Pharmacology Principles

Roadside Assistance

Pharmacology Principles
Roadside Assistance

Alan P. Agins, Ph.D.
Adjunct Associate Professor
Brown Medical School, Providence, Rhode Island
President, PRN Associates
Continuing Healthcare Education
Tucson, Arizona

Workbook prepared by

Kathleen Jo Gutierrez, Ph.D.,
RN, ANP-BC, CNS-BC
Independent Practice, Littleton, Colorado
Associate Professor School of Nursing
University of Colorado at Denver Health Sciences Center
Denver, Colorado

MOSBY

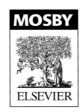

ELSEVIER

11830 Westline Industrial Drive
St. Louis, Missouri 63146

PHARMACOLOGY PRINCIPLES: ROADSIDE ASSISTANCE   ISBN: 978-0-323-04415-8
Copyright © 2007 by Mosby, Inc., an affiliate of Elsevier Inc.

Notice

Knowledge and best practice in this field are constantly changing. As new research and experience broaden our knowledge, changes in practice, treatment, and drug therapy may become necessary or appropriate. Readers are advised to check the most current information provided (i) on procedures featured or (ii) by the manufacturer of each product to be administered, to verify the recommended dose or formula, the method and duration of administration, and contraindications. It is the responsibility of the practitioner, relying on their own experience and knowledge of the patient, to make diagnoses, to determine dosages and the best treatment for each individual patient, and to take all appropriate safety precautions. To the fullest extent of the law, neither the Publisher nor the Authors assumes any liability for any injury and/or damage to persons or property arising out or related to any use of the material contained in this book.

The Publisher

Note from the author:
The appearance of a specific brand name drug does not constitute an endorsement of that product by the authors.

ISBN: 978-0-323-04415-8

Acquisitions Editor: Kristin Geen
Developmental Editor: Jamie Horn
Editorial Assistant: Jennifer Stoces
Book Production Manager: Gayle May
Project Manager: Tracey Schriefer
Design Direction: Paula Ruckenbrod
Cover Design Direction: Paula Ruckenbrod

Printed in China

Last digit is the print number: 9   8   7   6   5   4   3   2   1

Working together to grow
libraries in developing countries

www.elsevier.com | www.bookaid.org | www.sabre.org

ELSEVIER   BOOK AID International   Sabre Foundation

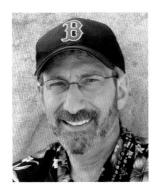

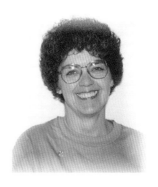

Alan P. Agins, PhD, is a pharmacologist who has lectured nationally since 1995 to more than 40,000 advanced practice clinicians, including nurses, nurse practitioners, physicians, physician assistants, pharmacists, dentists and other allied healthcare professionals. Dr. Agins received his Bachelor of Science degree in psychology from the State University of New York (Brockport). He received a master's degree in pharmacology and toxicology and his PhD in pharmaceutical sciences from the University of Rhode Island.

Dr. Agins has held faculty appointments at Brown Medical School, Northeastern University School of Pharmacy, and University of Virginia School of Nursing, and has also taught graduate/postgraduate pharmacology courses for a number of nursing schools around the country, including Pennsylvania State University, Idaho State University, Radford University, University of West Virginia, and University of Arizona. He currently holds an adjunct associate professorship in the medical school at Brown University, where he had been the recipient of the Dean's Teaching Excellence Award for four consecutive years (2001-2005).

Dr. Agins has been a regular presenter at the meetings of many national, regional, and state nurse practitioner organizations, and other professional nursing organizations; has provided keynote addresses at many conferences; and was an invited speaker for the Science, Technology, and Business Division of the Library of Congress in 2004.

He has written a book, *Parent and Educators Drug Reference* (PRN Press), and has written or co-authored journal articles, continuing education monographs, textbook chapters, and newsletters.

Dr. Agins has been widely praised by students, college administrators, healthcare professionals, and conference organizers for his wit and sense of humor, his ability to breathe life into dry subject matter, and his talent for using simple metaphors and analogies to make difficult concepts easy to grasp.

Kathleen Jo Gutierrez, PhD, completed an associate degree in nursing from the Community College of Denver, a Bachelor of Science degree in nursing from Metropolitan State College of Denver, and a Master of Science degree from the University of Colorado at Denver Health Sciences Center. She also completed a post-master's program as an adult nurse practitioner through Beth El College in Colorado Springs. Her interest in education and professional development led her to a doctoral degree in education from the University of Denver.

Dr. Gutierrez is a primary health care provider in the Denver area. In the 20 years before entering private practice, she was an associate professor of nursing at Regis University in Denver and is presently an associate professor with the University of Colorado at Denver Health Sciences Center.

In addition to her work on *Saunders Nursing Survival Guide: Pathophysiology*, Dr. Gutierrez is the author and editor of *Pharmacotherapeutics: Clinical Reasoning in Practice*, *Pharmacotherapeutics: Clinical Decision-Making in Nursing*, and *Pharmacology for Nursing Practice*, and co-author of *Saunders Nursing Survival Guide: Pharmacology*.

Dr. Gutierrez is named in *Who's Who in American Nursing*, *Who's Who in American Education*, *Who's Who in Medicine and Health Care*, and most recently, *Who's Who in American Women*. She is board certified as both an adult nurse practitioner and medical-surgical clinical nurse specialist. She is a member of the American Nurses Association, National Organization of Nurse Practitioner Faculties, American Academy of Nurse Practitioners, American Association of Diabetes Educators, and Sigma Theta Tau International, Honour Society of Nursing.

Reviewers

DIANE BENSON, RN, EDD
Associate Professor and Chair
Department of Nursing
Humboldt State University
Arcata, California

DARLENE CLARK, RN, MS
Senior Lecturer in Nursing
Penn State University School of Nursing
University Park, Pennsylvania

KATHLEEN M. GEIB, DNSC, CNS, RN
Assistant Professor
College of Nursing
Kent State University
Kent, Ohio

SHERRY NEELY, MSN, RN, CRNP
Associate Professor
Nursing and Allied Health
Butler County Community College

DEBRA PEYTON, MSN, RN
Assistant Professor of Nursing
Allen College
Waterloo, Iowa

Pharmacology Principles | Roadside Assistance

How to use your workbook and DVD

This workbook/DVD package provides many features that will make learning pharmacology a breeze. By reviewing the engaging and humorous videos and using the workbook modules as a study and review tool, you will be able to make sense of key pharmacology concepts almost effortlessly and have fun at the same time. Take a minute to familiarize yourself with the format so you get the most out of this exciting product!

The workbook features 10 modules covering essential pharmacology principles. The format for these modules is outlined below. Remember: each workbook module is accompanied by a presentation on the DVD.

WORKBOOK FORMAT

Each module in the workbook should be completed as follows:

How Long?

This section allows you to estimate how much time you will need to complete the module.

Content Overview

Here you will find an introduction to the topic and an explanation of related concepts. Key terms are in boldface to highlight important words and ideas. This brief overview of content serves as a foundation for the video clips.

Points to Remember

Review this list of key concepts to solidify your understanding of concepts introduced in the Content Overview.

For Your Viewing Pleasure

When you reach this section, you are ready to view the corresponding module on the DVD. Pop the disc into a DVD player, sit back, and enjoy the show!

Learning Activities

Now that you have reviewed all the necessary material, you are ready to put that knowledge into practice. Complete various activities, such as labeling, filling in the blanks, reviewing terminology, doing crossword puzzles, and more!

Test Your Knowledge

Wrap it all up by answering the quiz questions in this section and seeing how much information you recall from the material you have just studied. Bonus: this section has a special icon that indicates questions in NCLEX format.

An answer key is included in the back of the workbook for you to check answers for the Learning Activities and Test Your Knowledge sections. A glossary of key terms is also included at the end of the workbook.

Be sure to review this workbook and DVD as often as necessary to be sure you have a solid understanding of this essential information. Have fun and good luck!

Table of Contents

Module 1

Pharmacology: Speaking the Language

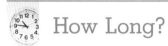 How Long?

Video: Approximately 3 minutes
Workbook: Approximately 60 minutes

 Content Overview

This module presents the basic principles of pharmacology upon which drug therapy is based. **Pharmacotherapeutics** is the use of drugs to alleviate the signs and symptoms of disease, delay disease progression, cure a disease, or facilitate nondrug interventions. Whenever a drug is used, the benefits of its use should be greater than the risks of side effects. All aspects of the use of a drug must be considered.

Pharmacology is the study of the mechanism of action, uses, side effects, and fate of drugs in the body. In other words, it is the study of what biologically active compounds do in the body **(pharmacodynamics),** and how the body reacts to them **(pharmacokinetics).** There are thousands of drugs and hundreds of facts about each one. Memorizing facts is unnecessary if you can predict the behavior of each drug based on a few facts and an understanding of the principles of pharmacology.

Today, most drugs are synthetic in origin; they are discovered and compounded in a laboratory although a few are still obtained from natural sources. The name given a new drug is almost as important as the drug itself. Systematic study of pharmacology requires the use of standardized language. A drug usually has three names a generic name, one that is simpler than the chemical name and identifies or classifies the drug in scientific literature; and a brand name, or trade name, which identifies the drug as the product of a specific manufacturer. Some examples are shown in the following table.

Chemical Name	Generic Name	Brand/Trade Name
N-acetyl-para-aminophenol	acetaminophen	Tylenol
Acetylsalicylic acid	aspirin	Bufferin
7-chloro-1,3-dihydro-1-methyl-5-phenyl-2H-1,4-benzodiazepin-2-one	diazepam	Valium
1-methyl-4-phenylisonipecotate hydrochloride	meperidine	Demerol
17,21-dihydroxypregna-1,4-diene-3,11,20-trione	prednisone	Deltasone

As you can see, **chemical names** are based on the drug's precise chemical structure, which conform to a specific set of international rules. These names are complex and therefore not practical for everyday use. The **generic name** of a drug is simpler than the chemical name and identifies or classifies the drug in scientific literature. All prescription drugs and many over-the-counter (OTC) drugs have a single generic name. The generic name of a drug is assigned by the United States Adopted Name (USAN) Council, in consultation with the pharmaceutical company developing the drug. The purpose of the United States Adopted Names (USAN) Council is to serve the health professions in the United States by selecting simple, informative, and unique nonproprietary drug names by establishing logical nomenclature classifications based on pharmacological and/or chemical relationships.

The USAN Council (tri-sponsored by the American Medical Association [AMA], the United States Pharmacopeial Convention [USP], and the American Pharmacists Association [APhA]) strives for global standardization and unification of drug nomenclature and related rules to ensure that drug information is accurately and unambiguously communicated. The USAN works closely with the International Nonproprietary Name (INN) Programme of the World Health Organization (WHO), and various national nomenclature groups.

Manufacturers assign a drug's **brand or trade name,** which is copyrighted by the pharmaceutical company and is legally on record for 20 years. Pharmaceutical companies want names that are easily recognized and easily pronounced by patients and health care providers. Unfortunately, having multiple brand names for a single generic drug may complicate recognition of the drug and increases the possibility of drug errors. For example, the generic drug ibuprofen is sold under the brand names Advil, Motrin, Nuprin, Genpril, Q-Profen, as well as under many store brand names. This is why it is important to know and use the generic name. It helps to avoid confusion and reduces the risk of duplication in patient treatment regimens.

As more drugs enter the marketplace, health care providers, pharmacists, and the public are often bewildered by subtle differences in spelling. Between 1998 and 2004, more than 60 new sound-alike drug names were introduced. Sometimes the similarities in name caused errors that were detrimental to patients. Most drug errors occurred when the drug name was similar to that of a more frequently prescribed product; it could be misread, misheard, or miswritten (see Module 6).

Because no organization is addressing the problem of sound-alike trade names, health care providers and their patients must become familiar with the name and appearance of a drug, and the disorder for which a drug is prescribed. When a new prescription is filled, the drug name should be checked and the pharmacist notified of the reason the drug was prescribed.

The need for objective, concise, well-organized information on drugs is obvious. However, there is no single source of drug information that covers all clinical situations. Resources include pharmacology and therapeutic textbooks, professional journals, drug compendia, continuing education seminars and meetings, advertising, drug information centers, and online computer databases.

The only official book of drug standards in the United States is *The United States Pharmacopeia/National Formulary* (USP–NF), a privately issued compendium first published in 1820. The USP–NF is published annually with one main addition and two supplements. The current edition of USP–NF is the only official edition. For the purpose of law within the United States, it is important to establish compliance with standards and procedures in the current official edition. Older editions are not acceptable for official compliance. For example, USP 29–NF 24, which became official on January 1, 2006, features significant new information since the previous edition, USP 28–NF 23. The new 2006 edition has nearly 500 new

and revised monographs and 40 new and revised general chapters. Drugs included in the reference meet high standards of quality, purity, and strength, and are identified by the letters USP–NF following the official name.

Points to Remember

• Use the generic name of a drug when possible. It helps to avoid confusion and reduces the risk of duplication in patient treatment regimens.

• If a brand name must be used, also include the generic name. Drugs coming from other countries have the same generic name but different brand names.

• Inevitably, situations occur in which needed drug information is not contained in available resources. The health care provider may consult with a pharmacist or use an online drug database.

For Your Viewing Pleasure

Now check out the video clip for Module 1 on your CD.

Learning Activities

Anagrams

Unscramble the anagrams below to find terms related to drugs and drug therapy

1. I a checkpoints arm

_____

2. conspiracy dam ham

_____

3. my car pool hag

_____

4. eminence rag

_____

5. bad men ran

_____

Fill in the Blanks

6. The only official book of drug standards is the
_____.

7. Having multiple _____ names for a single
generic drug impairs _____ of the drug
and increases the possibility of _____
_____.

8. The generic name of a drug is assigned by the
United States _____ _____ Council, in
consultation with the _____
company developing the drug.

9. Whenever a drug is used, the _____ of its
use should be greater than the _____ of side
effects.

10. _____ is the study of what
biologically active compounds do in the body.

Word Finding

**Circle the words in the puzzle below that
relate to pharmacotherapeutics.**

AMA	Official
Book	OTC
Brand name	Pharmacist
Chemical name	Pharmacokinetics
Drug error	Pharmacology
Generic name	Prescription
Nurse	

```
A  B  C  D  E  F  G  H  I  J  K  L  M  L  N  O  P
V  P  E  D  C  B  T  S  I  C  A  M  R  A  H  P  Q
G  H  H  I  J  K  L  Z  Y  X  W  V  U  I  W  E  R
M  A  N  A  O  P  Q  R  S  T  A  U  V  C  W  X  Y
D  R  C  B  R  A  N  D  N  A  M  E  D  I  B  Q  Z
E  M  F  G  H  M  I  J  K  L  A  M  N  F  O  P  Q
S  A  R  T  Y  U  A  I  O  P  M  B  C  F  X  V  Z
F  C  D  P  R  E  S  C  R  I  P  T  I  O  N  S  A
G  O  H  J  K  L  M  E  O  T  N  B  V  C  X  Z  Q
H  K  J  K  L  P  O  S  I  L  U  Y  T  R  E  R  W
G  I  F  D  S  A  Z  R  X  C  O  V  B  K  O  O  B
A  N  B  C  D  E  F  U  G  H  I  G  J  K  L  R  M
G  E  N  E  R  I  C  N  A  M  E  Q  Y  P  O  R  N
R  T  S  T  U  J  B  X  C  N  K  U  A  S  D  E  F
G  I  H  J  K  L  Z  V  X  N  F  G  J  U  Y  G  R
L  C  H  E  M  I  C  A  L  N  A  M  E  E  R  U  L
M  S  P  R  T  V  T  X  Z  L  K  J  H  G  F  R  F
N  O  Q  S  U  W  O  Y  A  S  D  F  G  H  J  D  K
```

Test Your Knowledge

Directions: Circle the best response.

1. The study of how drugs enter the body, reach the site of action, and are removed from the body is called:
   1. Pharmacotherapeutics
   2. Pharmacology
   3. Pharmacodynamics
   4. Pharmacokinetics

2. The use of generic drug names is recommended because:
   1. They can then be classified in published literature
   2. They are easily recognized and pronounced
   3. They identify the drug's precise chemical structure
   4. They are used when writing prescriptions

3. Manufacturers of brand name drugs hold the drug's name copyright for:
   1. 7 years
   2. 10 years
   3. 13 years
   4. 20 years

4. Chemical names of drugs:
   1. Are easily recognized and pronounced
   2. Allow the drug to be classified in published literature
   3. Are used when writing prescriptions
   4. Identify the drug's precise chemical structure

5. The brand name of a drug:
   1. Allows the drug to be classified in published literature
   2. Identifies the drugs precise chemical structure
   3. Identifies the drug as coming from a specific manufacturer
   4. Means it is a higher quality drug than a generic drug

Answer Key

Module 1
Pharmacology: Speaking the Language

LEARNING ACTIVITIES
Anagrams
1. Pharmacokinetics
2. Pharmacodynamics

3. Pharmacology
4. Generic name
5. Brand name

Fill in the Blanks
6. U.S. Pharmacopeia
7. Brand; recognition; drug errors
8. Adopted Name; pharmaceutical
9. Benefits; risks
10. Pharmacodynamics

Word Finder

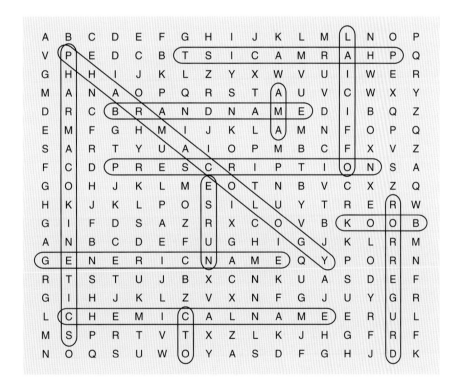

TEST YOUR KNOWLEDGE
1. 2
2. 1
3. 4
4. 4
5. 3

Module 2

Know Your Rights

 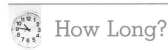 How Long?

Video: Approximately 3 minutes
Workbook: Approximately 60 minutes

Content Overview

When it comes to pharmacotherapy the nurse needs to know and understand all of the information about the patient and each medication prescribed. Medication errors can occur at any point in providing drugs to patients, including selecting, procuring, storing, prescribing, ordering, filling an order, preparing, dispensing, administering, monitoring, and documenting. That is why it is so critical for the nurse to always adhere to the "five rights of medication administration": right drug, right dose, right patient, right route, and right time. Sometimes sixth and seventh rights are included: the right documentation and the right to refuse the drug.

RIGHT DRUG

When a drug is first ordered, the nurse compares the medication record or computer orders with the health care provider's written orders. When administering the drug the nurse compares the label of the drug container with the medication record. Such checking is done three times: (1) before removing the container from the drawer or shelf; (2) as the amount of drug prescribed is removed from the container, and (3) before returning the container to storage. If the drug is unfamiliar, seek information from an authoritative source. Read labels of drug containers accurately. Question the prescribing health care provider about the order if it is unclear or if the drug seems inappropriate for the patient's age or condition.

RIGHT DOSE

The unit dose system is designed to minimize errors. When a drug must be prepared from a larger volume or strength, or when the health care provider orders a system of measurement different from what the pharmacist supplies, the chance of error increases. When it is necessary to calculate a dose, the nurse should have another qualified nurse check the calculated dose. However, in some situations this may not be feasible. The professional nurse should be able to accurately double-check her or his calculation by reversing the math.

Be sure to measure doses accurately using standard measuring devices, such as graduated medicine cups, syringes, and scaled droppers. A scored tablet may be cut in half by using a knife-edge or a cutting device. Tablet crushing devices should be cleaned completely before crushing a drug. Remember though, not all drugs can or should be crushed. Time-released, sustained-release, or extended-release formulations have special coatings or are formulated in such a fashion as to prevent the drug from being absorbed too quickly.

RIGHT PATIENT

Drug errors often occur because one patient gets a drug intended for another patient. An important step in drug administration is to be sure the drug is given to the right patient. In many cases, it is after a patient transfer or the discharge of patients that many drug errors occur.

A simple yet effective way to avoid mix-ups is to always ask the patient to state his or her name prior to administering the drug, and to check the patient's identification (ID) band against the medication administration record. If an ID bracelet becomes smudged or illegible, or is missing, the nurse must acquire a new one for the patient before giving the drug. These steps are not time-consuming, and they are easy to implement and explain to nursing staff. If they are followed, the chances of a patient receiving a drug intended for another patient are all but zero.

RIGHT ROUTE

This is an issue of how the drug is to be administered. Does the pharmacy check the order to make sure it is indicated for the right route—by mouth, inhalation, IV infusion, etc.? Is the route clearly identified on the pharmacy label for the person administering the drug? Consult with the health care provider if the drug order does not include a route of administration. Prepare injections only from formulations designed for parenteral use. Drug manufacturers label parenteral drugs "for injectable use only." The injection of a liquid or suspension designed for oral use can produce local complications, such as sterile abscesses, or produce fatal systemic effects.

RIGHT TIME

The nurse must know why a drug is ordered for certain times of the day and whether that schedule can be altered. Each health care institution has a recommended time schedule for drug administration, although the schedule can sometimes be altered based on patient needs. Schedule drug administration to maximize therapeutic effects and minimize adverse effects. All routine drugs should be administered within 60 minutes of the time ordered (30 minutes before or after the prescribed time). There is a tendency to over-rely on prescribed schedules. Establish a drug administration routine with standardized times. Place clearly visible reminders, such as large clocks, in places where nurses can see them. When the patient is transferred from area to area, make sure clear instructions regarding medication administration accompany him or her. The receiving nurse must be informed of what has been—or has yet to be—given to the patient.

RIGHT DOCUMENTATION

This right has been added to the five rights of medication administration by several authors to improve medication administration safety. Medication errors can result from inaccurate documentation. Documentation of drug administration should clearly include the patient's name, name of the drug ordered, the time given, and the drug's dosage, route, and frequency. Complete the medication administration

record immediately after giving the drug according to agency policy, and verify that the drug was given as ordered. Accurate documentation serves as a means for health care providers to communicate with each other. Additionally, ensure accuracy once per day by verifying the original drug order with the records used for preparation and administration of the drug.

RIGHT TO REFUSE

This right is also added to the five rights of medication administration by authors who focus on patient rights. Even though the health care provider has written the order, the pharmacy has filled the medicine boxes, and the nurse has prepared the drug for administration, the patient has a right to refuse to take it. This assumes, of course, that the patient is coherent and understands the implications of such action. It is important to document the patient's refusal, the reason for the refusal, and the notification of the health care provider.

 Points to Remember

- Check for patient allergies before administering any drug.

- Use sound nursing judgment in collaboration with pharmacy personnel while following agency policy regarding drug administration regimens.

- Teach the patient the drug's name, purpose, action, and potential undesired effects. In addition, confirm that the patient (and/or family member) understands this information and agrees to take the drug. Informed consent is determined by the nursing assessment or evaluation of the patient's knowledge, not by just talking with the appropriate health care provider.

- It is the nurse's professional responsibility to check the order and the label on the medication container, and to check for *all* of the five rights at least three times prior to giving the drug to the patient.

 For Your Viewing Pleasure

Now check out the video clip for Module 2 on your CD.

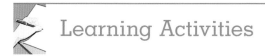
Learning Activities

What is Wrong with this Picture?

In the following scenarios, identify the actions the nurse would take to reduce the risk of violating a patient's five rights.

1. You enter a patient's room to administer medications at 9 AM. You hear the shower running and see that his name band is on the bedside table.

2. Hospital policy states that drugs to be administered twice daily should be given at 9 AM and 5 PM. The patient insists that the second dose of the day be administered at 9 PM.

3. When checking the order against the chart you find that an unusually large dosage has been ordered.

4. You find that multiple tablets are needed to prepare the ordered dose.

5. The health care provider calls the nursing unit to leave pain medication orders for the new patient.

Matching

Complete the statement in Column A with the remainder of the statement in Column B

Column A

6. The first check in making sure the "right drug" is being prepared is done

7. The second check in making sure the "right drug" is being prepared is done

8. The third check in making sure the "right drug" is being prepared is done

9. When calculating a dose of medication the nurse should

10. Drug manufacturers label parenteral drugs

Column B

A. before returning the medication to storage.

B. before removing the medication from the dispenser.

C. after the patient's name band is checked.

D. for injectable use only.

E. have the calculations checked by another nurse before giving the medication.

F. as the medication is removed from the container.

Crossword Puzzle

Complete the crossword puzzle regarding patient rights.

Across

3. Which one?
4. Who?
5. How?

Down

1. Nurses responsibility
2. Patient's right
3. When?
4. How much?

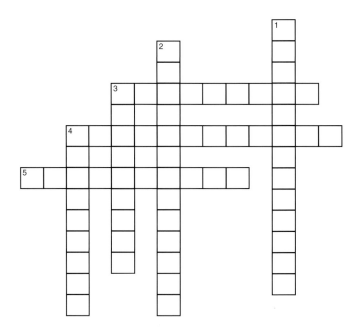

Test Your Knowledge

Directions: Circle the best response.

1. The nurse is having difficulty reading an order for a drug. The nurse knows the health care provider is very busy and does not like to be disturbed for such minor problems. The nurse should:

   1. Ask the unit secretary to interpret the physician's handwriting
   2. Call a pharmacist to interpret the orders
   3. Call the health care provider to have the order clarified
   4. Consult the unit manager to help interpret the orders

2. Which of the following rights has been added to the traditional five rights of medication administration?

   1. Right time
   2. Right route
   3. Right drug
   4. Right documentation

3. Which of the components of the drug order identified below is missing? There may be more than one correct answer.

   6-15-06   azithromycin 500 mg today then
              250 mg daily for 4 days.

   _____
   _____
   _____

4. Is the following drug order complete as it is written?

   October 18, 1990—2 p.m.

   Beclomethasone inhaled 40 mcg/spray

   Use 1 to 2 sprays in each nostril twice daily

   Dr. Howard Khnowitaally

   _____Yes

   _____No

5. Documentation of drug administration should clearly reflect the _____ name, name of the _____ administered, the _____ given, and the drug's _____, _____, and _____.

Answer Key

Module 2
Know Your Rights

LEARNING ACTIVITIES
What is Wrong with this Picture?

1. Wait until the patient completes his shower and arrange for a replacement arm band before administering the patient's medications.

2. Review hospital policy. Ask the patient the reason for his request. Check to be sure the drug can be safely administered at 9 PM. Notify the health care provider of the request. If appropriate, note the change in administration time in the medication record and the patient record.

3. Check the drug's usual dosage range in an official reference, or contact pharmacy personnel for clarification. If the dose is excessive, notify the health care provider of the normal dosage range; ask for a change in the medication order.

4. Clarify the available formulations with pharmacy personnel. If correct, administer the drug. If incorrect, contact the health care provider for clarification of the order.

5. Obtain a thorough patient history and information about allergies. Assess patient pain level before administering pain medication.

Matching

6. B
7. F
8. A
9. E
10. D

Crossword Puzzle
Across
3. Right drug
4. Right patient
5. Right route
Down
1. Documentation
2. Right to refuse
3. Right time
4. Right dose

TEST YOUR KNOWLEDGE
1. 3
2. 4
3. Patient name, route, purpose for the drug
4. No, missing patient name
5. Patient's; drug; time; dosage; route; frequency

Module 3

Pharmacokinetics I

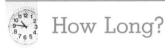 How Long?

Video: Approximately 10 minutes
Workbook: Approximately 60 minutes

 Content Overview

PHARMACEUTICAL PHASE

Drug activity occurs in three phases: the pharmaceutic phase, the pharmacokinetic phase, and the pharmacodynamic phase. The **pharmaceutic phase** of drug activity begins with the manufacturer's formulating drugs into dosage forms that are suitable for delivery into the patient. The pharmaceutic phase also describes the processes that occur when the drug enters the body in one form, say a tablet, and changes to another form (individual drug molecules) so that it can get into the system and exert an action.

Active ingredients are responsible for producing desired effects and vary considerably in their chemical structure. The major classes of active ingredients include alkaloids, glycosides, polypeptides, organic salts, and steroids. Additives may be used to alter certain properties of the final drug formulation. They typically consist of binders, diluents, disintegrators, dyes, flavorings, fillers, and vehicles. They must be nontoxic and compatible with the active ingredient as well as with each of the additives.

Drug **formulations** are designed and administered to produce either local or systemic effects. Formulations for local use come in many forms, including aerosols, ointments, creams, pastes, powders, tinctures, and lotions. They can also be formulated as gels, foams, and suppositories for rectal, vaginal, or urethral use. Drugs can also be formulated as a douche (i.e., vaginal irrigation) or as an enema (i.e., rectal irrigation). Sprays, aerosols, gases, and nebulizers are methods of introducing drugs to the respiratory system for either local or systemic effects or both.

Systemic drug formulations are designed for oral, topical, or parenteral use. **Parenteral** drugs are introduced into the body by any route other than enteral. These include injectable solutions delivered by intravenous (IV), intramuscular (IM), subcutaneous or intrathecal routes. Ointments, pastes, or patches placed on the skin (topical) can also be used to provide systemic levels of certain drugs. **Enteral** administration includes delivery of drugs by oral, sublingual, buccal, or rectal routes. Delivery of drugs into the gastrointestinal tract by gastric (G) or nasogastric (NG) tubes is also considered enteral administration. Drugs for enteral administration may be formulated as tablets, capsules, lozenges, liquid suspensions or solutions.

PHARMACOKINETIC PHASE

Pharmacokinetics is the science of how the body handles the chemicals (drugs) we put into it. The processes of absorption, distribution, metabolism, and elimination ultimately determine the disposition and fate of drugs in the body over a period of time. In other words, pharmacokinetics is "what the body does to the drug."

Absorption

Absorption is defined as the movement of a drug from the administration site to the systemic circulation (e.g., from the stomach to the circulation; from the muscle to the circulation). Absorption is needed for a drug to produce a pharmacologic action. Factors influencing the rate and extent of drug absorption into the circulation include dosage form, administration route, age of patient, and disease states. The rate at which drugs are absorbed determines the onset of effects. In turn, the amount of drug absorbed determines the magnitude of effects. In many cases, drug absorption uses the same pathways as nutrients. **Passive diffusion** is the process that moves drugs from an area of higher concentration (e.g., the intestine) to an area of lower concentration (e.g., the circulation) across a semipermeable membrane (the intestinal wall). This mechanism accounts for the absorption of most drugs from the gastrointestinal (GI) tract into the circulation and from the circulation to target cells.

In some cases, especially when drug molecules are very large, **pinocytosis** facilitates drug absorption by engulfing those large molecules and moving them across cell membranes. During pinocytosis, the cell wall invaginates, forms a vacuole for drug transport, breaks off, and moves into the cell. Think of a Pac-Man when you see pinocytosis.

Active transport is a process that moves drug molecules against a concentration gradient, using metabolic energy in the form of adenosine triphosphate (ATP). The ATP-drug complex forms on the surface of the cell membrane, carries the drug through the membrane, and then dissociates on the other side. In this case, think of an automatic revolving door at a hotel. The rate of active transport is proportional to drug concentration.

The **molecular size** of a drug plays a part in drug absorption. For example, small molecules like aspirin, morphine, or propranolol can easily pass across cell membranes. Once the concentrations on both sides of the cell membrane are equal, drug movement stops. In contrast, heparin molecules or proteins like insulin are too large and do not pass across cell membranes. These drugs need to circumvent cell membranes by being injected.

To pass through membranes lining the gastrointestinal tract, a drug must be relatively fat, or **lipid soluble,** because the membranes of the cells themselves contain a high concentration of lipid. In that regard, the movement of a drug across membranes by passive diffusion can be influenced by the electrical charge **(polarity)** of the drug molecule. Some drugs are weak organic acids, some are weak organic bases, and some are simply neutral. Nonionized (nonpolar) drug molecules are usually lipid soluble and capable of crossing cell membranes. In contrast, drug molecules that are ionized (polar) are water soluble and thus unable to penetrate the fatty cell membranes.

Both the dissolution and relative degree of ionization of drugs are affected by the **pH** of body solutions. Remember, the pH of the stomach is acidic; the pH of the intestine is more alkaline. A good rule of thumb

is that acidic drugs, such as aspirin and ibuprofen, are nonionized in an acidic environment and thus are readily available for absorption in the acidic stomach. In contrast, basic drugs, such as morphine, certain antidepressants, and antihistamines, are more likely to be ionized in the acidity of the stomach and thus not readily absorbed until they reach the alkaline environment of the small intestines where they would become nonionized and absorbable.

In summary, small, lipid-soluble, nonionized drugs readily diffuse across cell membranes, whereas larger, water-soluble, ionized drugs do not.

Distribution

Once a drug has been absorbed (or injected), it enters the **distribution** phase. Distribution simply means that the drug is transported via the circulation to its site of action. Several factors influence the distribution of an absorbed drug, including the fat or water solubility of the drug and the amount of body fat or body water, the rate or extent of blood flow to the tissues, non-specific binding non-target tissue sites and binding to plasma proteins like albumin. Many drugs are bound to albumin, some with a high affinity. In some cases, as much as 99% of a drug in circulation is bound to albumin. Since albumin is such a large protein, it normally cannot get out of the blood vessel, nor can the drug molecules bound to it. Thus, only the fraction of drug that is not bound (free drug) is capable of leaving the blood vessel to get to its site of action in the tissues. The protein-bound drug is retained within the vessel and hence has no pharmacologic action. The effect is temporary, however, because as the unbound (free) drug leaves the circulation or is eliminated, bound drug is released from the protein binding site(s) in order to maintain an equilibrium between bound and free drug.

This becomes important in some cases. For example, if we give a drug that is normally highly protein-bound, but the patient has low albumin levels, the amount of drug that will now be free and capable of leaving the circulation to get to the target tissues may be too high and cause side effects or toxicity.

Metabolism

Drug Metabolism is the body's way to get rid of lipid-soluble drugs by transforming them into more water-soluble compounds, so they can be eliminated through the kidneys in urine. The enzymes that do this work are known as the cytochrome P450 microsomal enzymes and are located primarily in the liver and intestinal wall, but there is also some cytochrome P450 in almost every other tissue in the body.

When a drug undergoes metabolism, the reaction usually alters the chemical structure such that the metabolite is more water soluble than the parent drug. Many times the change in chemical structure makes the drug unrecognizable by its receptor, and thus the metabolite becomes inactive. Other times the chemical change may not alter the drug's ability to interact with its receptors. Because this metabolite works much like the parent drug, we call it an **active metabolite**. A **prodrug** is a drug that is has no pharmacologic activity until it is metabolized; prodrugs must be metabolized in the body to become active. Finally, in some instances, a drug may be totally safe and effective, but it may be transformed into a **toxic metabolite**.

Elimination

Drug **elimination** refers to the movement of a drug or its metabolites from the tissues back into the circulation and then to the organs of elimination. The primary system responsible for drug elimination is the kidneys, but elimination also occurs to lesser degrees in the GI tract, respiratory system, sweat, saliva, tears, and breast milk. The kidneys use **glomerular filtration** and active tubular secretion to rid the body of unchanged, unbound drug molecules and their metabolites. Like sodium and potassium, drugs that are not bound to plasma proteins are filtered through the glomerulus to enter the urine. Clearly, the more water-soluble the drug or the metabolite, the more likely it will stay in the urine. **Passive reabsorption** takes place when a drug is nonionized and still has sufficient lipid solubility to diffuse back from the urine into the circulation. **Active transport** pumps may recognize certain acidic or basic drug molecules in efferent blood flow and secrete them across the brush border membranes into the proximal tubules. Despite this mechanism, if any of these three processes is faulty, such as the

creatinine, clearance rate is too low, or the serum creatinine levels are too high, the doses of certain drugs need to be reduced to prevent side effects and toxicity.

Points to Remember

- Drug absorption is influenced by pH; acidic drugs are nonionized in an acidic environment; basic drugs are nonionized in an alkaline environment.

- High lipid solubility and low protein binding favor diffusion of a drug through membranes.

- Only free, unbound drugs are available to cross cell membranes to sites of action; a protein-bound drug has no pharmacologic action.

- Metabolism helps to rid the body of lipid-soluble drugs by transforming them into water-soluble compounds for elimination in urine.

- Drug elimination refers to the movement of a drug or its metabolites from the tissues back into the circulation and then to the organs of elimination (i.e., kidney).

For Your Viewing Pleasure

Now check out the video clip for Module 3 on your CD.

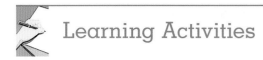 Learning Activities

Crossword Puzzle

Fill in the crossword puzzle using pharmacokinetic terminology.

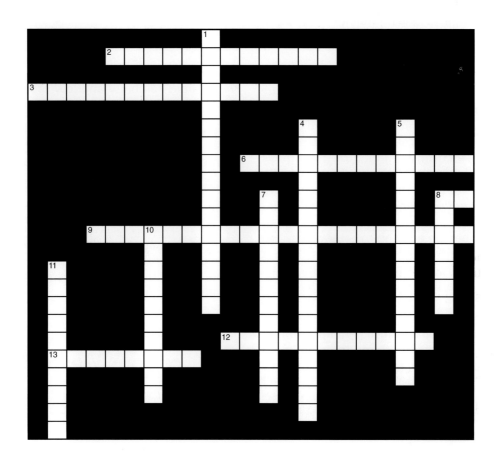

Across

2. Describes the stage during which the drug enters the body in one form and changes to another form to become active

3. One of the factors influencing movement of drugs across cell membranes

6. Movement of drug molecules from their site of absorption to their site of action

8. The alkalinity or acidity of a drug or body tissue

9. The process by which drugs enter the proximal tubules of the kidneys

12. Removal of drug molecules from the body

13. Refers to the ionization or nonionization of a drug

Down

1. Movement of drug molecules from areas of higher to lower concentration

4. The substances that produce drug activity

5. Moves drug molecules against a concentration gradient using metabolic energy in the form of ATP

7. The manufacturer makes these

8. A drug that must be metabolized before becoming active

10. The process of breaking a drug down into a water-soluble form

11. Movement of a drug from administration site to the blood stream

Fill in the Blanks

1. The _____ _____ of drug activity begins at the manufacturer with _____ drugs into dosage forms suited for delivery to the site of _____.

2. Active ingredients are responsible for producing _____ effects and vary considerably in their chemical structure.

3. _____ of the drug from its site of administration (e.g., skin, GI tract, muscle) into the blood stream is needed to produce pharmacologic effects.

4. For a drug to pass through membranes lining the gastrointestinal tract, a drug must be relatively _____ _____.

5. _____ drug molecules are usually _____ soluble and capable of crossing cell membranes. In contrast, _____ molecules are unable to penetrate lipid cell membranes.

6. Because only _____ drug is available to cross cell membranes to _____ _____ _____, the bound drug is lost to pharmacologic action.

7. The primary system responsible for drug elimination is the _____.

8. The kidneys use _____ _____ and active tubular secretion to rid the body of unchanged, unbound drug molecules and their metabolites.

True or False

If the answer is false, correct the statement to make it true.

1. _____ The pharmaceutic phase also describes the stage during which the drug enters the body in one form and changes to another form to become active.

2. _____ Drug formulations are designed and administered to produce either local or systemic effects.

3. _____ Active transport moves drugs from higher to lower concentrations across a semipermeable membrane.

4. _____ Small, lipid-soluble, nonionized drugs readily diffuse across cell membranes, whereas larger, water-soluble, ionized drugs do not.

5. _____ Basic drugs, such as aspirin and ibuprofen, are nonionized in an acidic environment and thus are readily available for absorption in the stomach.

6. _____ Acidic drugs, such as morphine and certain antidepressants, are more likely to be nonionized in the alkaline environment of the small intestines.

2. Which of the following ingredients in a drug would be considered an active ingredient rather than an additive?

1. Binder
2. Polypeptide
3. Dye
4. Filler

3. A patient is receiving supplemental doses of vitamin D, a lipid-soluble drug. The health care provider knows that this drug will be absorbed through which of the following mechanisms of transport?

1. Active transport
2. Filtration
3. Pinocytosis
4. Simple passive diffusion

4. When drugs undergo metabolism, the reaction usually alters the chemical structure of the drug so that its metabolite is more _____ _____ than the parent drug.

Test Your Knowledge

Directions: Circle the best response.

1. A health care provider would be particularly concerned about a patient's ability to adequately eliminate drugs that are prescribed if the patient had dysfunction of which of the following body systems?

1. Gastrointestinal
2. Cardiovascular
3. Renal
4. Respiratory

Answer Key

Module 3
Pharmacokinetics I

LEARNING ACTIVITIES

Crossword Puzzle
Across
 2. Pharmaceutic
 3. Molecular size
 6. Distribution
 8. pH
 9. Glomerular filtration
12. Elimination
13. Polarity
Down
 1. Passive diffusion
 4. Active ingredients
 5. Active transport
 7. Formulations
 8. Prodrug
10. Metabolism
11. Absorption

Fill in the Blanks
1. Pharmaceutic phase; formulating; action
2. Desired
3. Absorption
4. Lipid soluble
5. Nonionized (nonpolar); lipid; ionized (polar)
6. Free; sites of action
7. Kidneys
8. Glomerular filtration

True or False
1. True
2. True
3. False; passive diffusion
4. True
5. False; acidic drugs
6. False; basic drug

TEST YOUR KNOWLEDGE
1. 3
2. 2
3. 4
4. Water soluble

Module | 4

Pharmacokinetics II

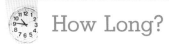 How Long?

Video: Approximately 5 minutes
Workbook: Approximately 60 minutes

 Content Overview

The route by which a drug is administered (e.g., oral, parenteral) affects how quickly it reaches a therapeutic blood level. However, while the actual dose of a drug and frequency of its administration determines the concentration of the drug in the plasma, these variables do not affect how long it takes that drug to reach **steady state**. Steady state refers to a plateau in the blood levels of a drug which occurs when the amount of drug being taken with each dose equals the amount of drug that lost by elimination from the body.

The term **half-life** ($t_{1/2}$) describes the relationship between plasma drug concentration and its steady state and clearance from the body. Half-life is defined as the time it takes for 50% of the drug in the body (at any time) to be eliminated. Half-life is an important variable in determining proper dosing and frequency of administration. The half-life of a given drug usually remains the same within each patient, assuming all elimination systems are functioning normally. For example, a patient arrives at an emergency room with a diagnosis of drug overdose. Assuming the patient's elimination systems are functioning and the elimination rate of the drug is not compromised, approximately 97% of the original dose will be eliminated after five half-lives, as follows:

- t_0 = time the drug is administered
- t_1 = 50% of the administered drug remains
- t_2 = 25% remains
- t_3 = 12.5% remains
- t_4 = 6.25% remains
- t_5 = 3.13% remains

A practical guide to the time it takes for a drug concentration to reach steady state can be obtained by multiplying the half-life by 5. This figure is very close to the time it will take to reach approximately 97% of the steady state value with continual dosing. The same holds true for drug elimination; multiply the half-life of the drug by 5 to obtain the length of time it will take the body to eliminate the drug once the drug is stopped.

The **onset of action** is the time it takes for an administered drug to begin eliciting an effect, such as analgesia or reduction in blood pressure. As the drug continues to be absorbed and distributed throughout the body, higher concentrations reach the site of action, and the effect increases in magnitude. The point at which drug is at its highest concentration and the therapeutic effect is at its maximum is known as the **peak effect**. If the peak level of a drug is too high, however, toxicity may result. Conversely, if the lowest blood level during the dosing interval (also known as the trough) is too low, then the drug may not be therapeutic. A drug's **duration of action** is the time from when the drug first produces its effect until that effect "wears off" or is no longer observable.

The kidneys eliminate many drugs from the body. Since most drugs are filtered from blood in the glomerulus, it is important to know the integrity of glomerular filtration. **Creatinine,** a normal by-product of muscle metabolism, is a chemical which is commonly used to assess glomerular function. Clinically, **creatinine clearance** (CrCL) is used to estimate the glomerular filtration rate (GFR) of the kidneys and thus the kidney's overall ability to eliminate drugs.

Normally, a drug with a high renal clearance is rapidly removed from the plasma and the patient may require more frequent dosing, higher doses of the drug, or both. Conversely, a drug that is slowly removed from the plasma in the kidneys has a low clearance rate and requires less frequent dosing. In that same context, if the kidneys are diseased or not working well, the clearance of many drugs may be reduced and thus may require dosage adjustments. Both clearance and half-life vary greatly from one drug to another.

1. _____ Drug absorption
2. _____ Drug concentration
3. _____ Drug elimination
4. _____ Therapeutic range
5. _____ Time
6. _____ Toxic range

Points to Remember

- Steady state refers to the plateau in drug levels in the blood when the amount of drug being taken is equal to the amount being eliminated.

- The terms *absorption, distribution, metabolism,* and *elimination* are used to describe the movement of drugs through the body. In contrast, the terms *onset, peak*, and *duration of action* are used to describe drug effects.

- A drug that is slowly removed from the plasma to be eliminated through the kidneys has a low clearance rate and requires less frequent dosing.

- A drug with a high renal clearance is rapidly removed from the plasma, thus requiring more frequent dosing and/or higher dosage of the drug.

- The term *half-life* describes the relationship between plasma concentrations of a drug and its clearance from the body.

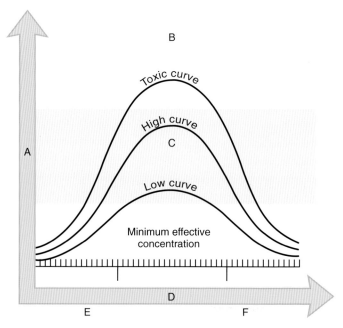

From Gutierrez K: Pharmacotherapeutics: clinical decision-making in nursing, Philadelphia, 1999, WB Saunders.

For Your Viewing Pleasure

Now check out the video clip for Module 4 on your CD.

Learning Activities

Dosing Curve

Identify the section of the dosing curve illustration on this page that best illustrates each of the following concepts.

Complete the Table

Complete the table on the next page by calculating the dosage of drug remaining in the body at each half-life, hours after peak concentration, and percentage of drug removed. The drug used in this example is one with a dose of 875 mg and a half-life of 12 hours.

Parameter	Changing Values					
Number of half-lives	t_0		t_2	t_3	t_4	t_5
Amount of drug remaining	875 mg					
Hours to peak concentration	0					
Percentage of drug removed	0					

Anagrams

Unscramble the anagram to find terms related to pharmacokinetics.

1. dye set tat as

   _____

2. fife hall

   _____

3. Inca foot notes

   _____

4. to turn aficionado

   _____

5. I a nice accent learner

   _____

 Test Your Knowledge

Directions: Circle the best response.

1. A health care provider uses knowledge of a drug's half-life as a factor in determining:

   1. The dosage and frequency of drug administration
   2. The precise timing of drug distribution
   3. The precise timing of drug elimination
   4. Which brand of a generic drug to mandate

2. The route by which a drug is administered affects how quickly it reaches its:

   1. Half-life
   2. Peak
   3. Onset of action
   4. Steady state

3. The _____ _____ _____ is the time it takes for a drug to begin eliciting a therapeutic response.

4. _____ describes the relationship between plasma drug concentration and its steady state and clearance from the body.

5. The time it takes for that drug to reach its highest effective concentration is known as the _____ _____.

6. A drug's _____ _____ _____ is the time it takes an effective drug concentration to elicit a therapeutic response.

7. You are caring for a 75-year-old female patient who is admitted for sepsis. The health care provider has added IV gentamicin every 12 hours to her treatment regimen, with instructions to obtain peak and trough levels with the third dose. The therapeutic range for gentamicin is 2 to 5 or 10 mcg/mL. The result for the patient's serum creatinine level has just arrived from the lab and it is 1.5 (normal for a female: 0.6-1.2 mg/dL). What information and nursing actions are required at this time to safely carry out the health care providers orders?

Answer Key

Module 4
Pharmacokinetics II

LEARNING ACTIVITIES
Dosing Curve

1. E
2. A
3. F
4. C
5. D
6. B

Complete the Table

Parameter	Values				
Number of half-lives	t_0	t_2	t_3	t_4	t_5
Amount of drug remaining (mg)*	875	437.5	218.7	109.3	54.6
Hours to peak concentration	0	12	24	36	48
Percentage of drug removed	0	50	75	88	94

*Answers for the amount of drug remaining do not total 875 mg because of rounding.

Anagram

1. Steady state
2. Half-life
3. Onset of action
4. Duration of action
5. Creatinine clearance

TEST YOUR KNOWLEDGE

1. 1
2. 4
3. Onset of action
4. Half-life
5. Peak effect
6. Duration of action
7. Determine what day and time the third dose is to be administered. Contact the health care provider for instructions regarding the patient's elevated serum creatinine level and the order for gentamicin. Plan to have the trough level of gentamicin drawn 30 to 60 minutes before administering the third dose and peak levels drawn 30 to 60 minutes after the IV infusion is complete. Monitor patient response.

Module 5

Pharmacodynamics

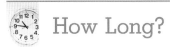

How Long?

Video: Approximately 6 minutes
Workbook: Approximately 60 minutes

Content Overview

The **pharmacodynamic phase** of drug activity occurs when a drug reaches its site of action and produces an effect; in other words, it is "where and how the drug acts in the body." The ability of a drug to bind to a specific receptor is determined by the chemical nature of the drug. This interaction is similar to a lock-and-key mechanism, where a critical portion of the drug determines its ability to bind. Drugs that differ in this critical region may not bind to the receptor at all.

The site of drug action is determined by many factors. A few drugs are administered so that they enter the body exactly where they are intended to act. Examples include antacids, which enter the stomach, dissolve, and neutralize excess stomach acid, and topical decongestants that are sprayed into the nostril to work directly in the nasal passages. Most drugs, however, must be absorbed or injected into the body where they eventually find their targets or receptors in the tissues.

In the body, chemicals such as neurotransmitters or hormones normally recognize and interact with specific receptors that are imbedded in the surface of cell membranes. These interactions, much like a key being put into a lock, serve normal physiologic or homeostatic functions. Drug molecules also recognize and interact with specific receptors in various tissues. Proteins within the cell membrane are the most common and important drug receptors and the binding of a drug molecule to its protein receptor is

reversible. It is known that a single receptor can react with a number of drugs, provided that each drug structurally conforms to the receptor site (the lock and key concept). Receptors are physiologic points of control. Theoretically, it should be possible to synthesize a drug that could alter any physiologic process for which receptors exist.

The majority of drugs act by attaching to receptors on cell surfaces. The actions that result from the binding include: (1) opening or closing ion channels; (2) activating biochemical messengers, such as cAMP or cGMP, which in turn initiate a series of chemical reactions within the cell; (3) inhibiting a cell from functioning too much as in a pathological state; or (4) turning on or increasing a normal cell's function.

How much of a drug is actually available in the body to produce an effect at the receptor site is known as its bioavailability. **Bioavailability** is a measure of how much of the drug actually gets into the body by any of the various routes of administration. Bioavailability is determined by cumulatively measuring drug concentration in body fluids (serum, urine, feces, etc.) over time. Bioavailability can be influenced by a number of things including the type of dosage form (tablets, capsules, suspensions, liquids, etc.), the presence of food within the GI tract, the type of foods or liquid consumed, or if a patient is fasting. The magnitude of a drug effect is directly proportional to the concentration of a drug at the receptor. The more drug, the more receptors occupied and the greater the pharmacological effect. Specificity is the property of receptors that allows them to differentiate between similar drugs and bind only to those with the critical features.

The ability to bind to the receptor and the capacity for stimulating an action by the receptor are two different aspects of drug action. The term **affinity** is used to describe the relative strength of a drug's binding to receptors. Drugs with a high affinity are strongly attracted to receptors and are generally considered potent drugs. For example, a 10-mg dose of morphine sulfate is equivalent to a 1-mg dose of hydromorphone. Therefore hydromorphone is the more potent drug. In other words, drugs with a great affinity for particular receptors are capable of eliciting a response at lower doses. The reverse is also true. Drugs with low affinity are less strongly attracted to receptors. They are generally weaker drugs that require large dosages to elicit a response.

Once a drug binds to a receptor there are essentially two possible outcomes. If the drug has **intrinsic activity,** the ability to activate the receptor, then a biological action will occur. For example, norepinephrine, naturally produced in nerve terminals, binds to specific proteins in arterial smooth muscle cells called $alpha_1$-adrenergic receptors. Stimulation of these receptors by norepinephrine causes vasoconstriction. Drugs that are similar in structure to norepinephrine can also bind to the $alpha_1$ receptors and cause a therapeutic "pressor" effect. Any compound, either natural or synthetic, that has affinity for a specific receptor and stimulates that receptor leading to a biological effect is called an **agonist**. In contrast, a drug that has an affinity for a receptor, but no intrinsic activity may not cause anything to happen. As long as the drug occupies the receptor site, however, other potential natural agonists are blocked from getting to that receptor. We call drugs like these **antagonists**. For example, the drug propranolol blocks $beta_1$-adrenergic receptors and prevents the natural agonist epinephrine (adrenalin) from stimulating the receptor. Propranolol therefore is classified as an antagonist to epinephrine. Antagonists are frequently called blockers or sometimes the prefix "anti" is used. In the example above, propranolol is known as a beta-**blocker.** In another example, diphenhydramine is an antagonist at $histamine_1$ receptors. Diphenhydramine is an "anti"histamine. Antagonists have an affinity for receptors but lack efficacy. When an antagonist occupies the receptor, the receptor cannot carry out its normal function.

Potency refers to the dosage needed to produce a response. The term "relative" potency is used to compare drugs within the same chemical class (e.g., opioids: morphine vs. fentanyl). Potency is influenced by the drug's affinity for receptors and by the body's absorptive, distributive, biotransformational, and elimination capabilities. **Efficacy,** on the other hand, refers to the degree to which a drug is able to produce its maximal effects. For example, if drug "A" (at its maximal dose) causes a 50-point drop in total cholesterol levels and drug "B" (at its maximal dose) produces a 20-point drop, drug "A" is the more efficacious. The term *efficacious* is used more easily, however, to compare drugs that have different mechanisms of action (e.g., analgesics: nonsteroidal antiinflammatory drugs vs. opioids).

Points to Remember

- Drugs do not create functions but modify existing functions within the body.

- No drug has a single action.

- When receptors are highly specific and have a high affinity for the drugs that bind to them, very small amounts of the drug can produce biologic activity.

- For a drug to be an agonist, it must have an affinity for a specific receptor, and it must display some degree of intrinsic activity.

- Potency is a measure of the dosage of a drug needed to produce a response.

- Antagonists have an affinity for receptors but lack intrinsic activity.

For Your Viewing Pleasure

Now check out the video clip for Module 5 on your CD.

Learning Activities

Anagrams

Unscramble the anagrams below to find terms related to the principles of drug action.

1. nations tag

_____

2. sit an go

_____

3. ceca iffy

_____

4. G man duet I

_____

5. anti iffy

_____

6. spec fit icy i

_____

7. srotpecer

_____

5. The term (affinity/potency) is used to describe the strength of a drug's binding to receptors.

6. (Efficacy/potency) refers to the degree to which a drug is able to produce maximal effects.

7. (Affinity/potency) refers to the dosage needed to produce a response.

8. Any compound, either natural or synthetic, that stimulates specific receptors is called an (agonist/antagonist).

Which Term is Correct?

Circle the term in the parentheses to make the statement correct.

1. Proteins of the cell membrane are the most important (drug receptors/drug agonists).

2. The (magnitude/specificity) of a drug effect is related to the effective concentration of the drug present at the receptor.

3. (Magnitude/specificity) is the property of receptors that allows them to differentiate among similar drugs and bind only to those with the critical features.

4. How much of a drug is actually available to produce an effect at the receptor is known as its (bioavailability/affinity).

Crossword Puzzle

Complete the diamond crossword by filling in terms related to pharmacodynamics. The numbers in parentheses identify the number of letters in each word.

Across

6. Relates to efficacy (7,7)

Down

1. When activated, these turn on a series of reactions within the cell (11,10)

2. Must be paired with an affinity for drug to be called an agonist (9,8)

3. Action of antagonist drug on an agonist drug (9)

4. Permit transfer of drugs across membranes (3,8)

5. Strength of a drug's binding to receptors (8)

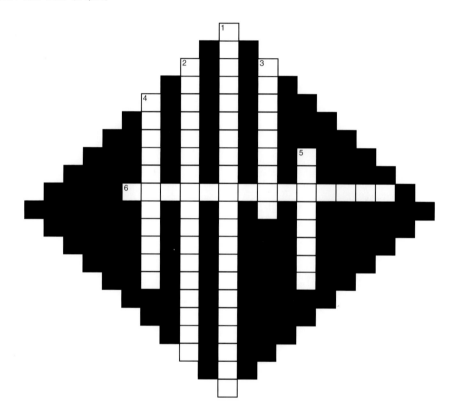

 Test Your Knowledge

Directions: Circle the best response.

1. A drug that mimics the effects of an endogenous chemical in the body is called a(n):

    1. Agonist
    2. Antagonist
    3. Competitive inhibitor
    4. Noncompetitive inhibitor

2. A health care provider is reading drug information pertaining to bioavailability. This term refers to which of the following properties of a drug?

    1. The ability of a drug to treat a disease or illness
    2. The concentration of the active drug in a specific drug preparation
    3. The degree to which a drug produces an effect through binding to its site of action
    4. The number and severity of adverse effects of a drug

3. The majority of drugs are thought to act by which of the following mechanisms?

   1. Altering protein synthesis inside the cell

   2. Attaching to receptors on the cell surface

   3. Changing the DNA structure within the cell

   4. Promoting cell growth

True or False

If the answer is false, correct the statement to make it true.

4. The specificity of a drug effect is related to the effective concentration of the drug present at the receptor.

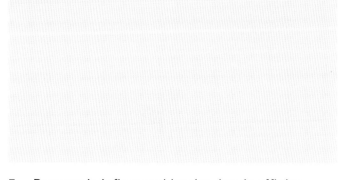

5. Potency is influenced by the drug's affinity for receptors and by the body's absorptive, distributive, metabolic, and elimination capabilities.

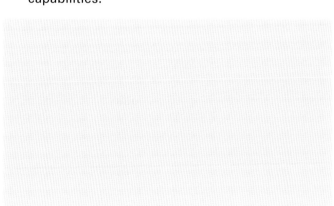

6. One drug that blocks the action of another drug at the receptor is known as an antagonist.

7. *Efficacy* refers to the degree to which a drug is able to produce maximal effects.

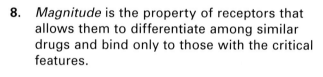

8. *Magnitude* is the property of receptors that allows them to differentiate among similar drugs and bind only to those with the critical features.

Answer Key

Module 5
Pharmacodynamics

LEARNING ACTIVITIES

Anagrams
1. Antagonist
2. Agonist
3. Efficacy
4. Magnitude
5. Affinity
6. Specificity
7. Receptors

Which Term is Correct?
1. Drug receptors
2. Magnitude
3. Specificity
4. Bioavailability
5. Affinity
6. Efficacy
7. Potency
8. Agonist

Crossword Puzzle

Across
6. Maximal effects.

Down
1. Biochemical messengers
2. Intrinsic activity
3. Inhibited
4. Ion channels
5. Affinity

TEST YOUR KNOWLEDGE
1. 1
2. 3
3. 2
4. False; the *magnitude* of drug effect is related to the effective concentration of the drug present at the receptor.
5. True
6. True
7. True
8. False; *specificity* is the property of receptors that allows them to differentiate among similar drugs and bind only to those with the critical features.

Module 6

Medication Errors

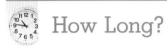

How Long?

Video: Approximately 6 minutes
Workbook: Approximately 60 minutes

Content Overview

A woman in the postanesthesia care unit (PACU) of a freestanding hospital is prescribed ondansteron (Zofran) for postoperative nausea. Unfortunately, the PACU nurse, who has been working a long shift and had her attention repeatedly diverted, hangs the wrong IV infusion bag without examining the label. The bag contains the common antibacterial drug metronidazole, which was intended to treat another patient's infection. The patient experiences vomiting, headaches, and abdominal cramps. Only later, when the nurse examines the IV bag more closely, does she recognize the mistake. Compounding the problem is that the printing on one bag looked very similar to the other.

If you think this could never happen in your facility, think again. Health care providers and insurance companies have become acutely aware of the real harm and monetary costs associated with medication errors and, as such, are taking steps to reduce such errors. According to the National Coordinating Council for Medical Error Reporting and Prevention (NCCMERP) (www.nccmerp.org), a medication error is defined as "any preventable event that may cause or lead to inappropriate medication use or patient harm while the medication is in the control of the health care professional, patient, or consumer". The council emphasizes finding problems in the medication handling system rather than assigning blame to individuals.

The NCCMERP includes such founding members as the American Association of Retired Persons (www.

aarp.org), the American Medical Association (www. ama-assn.org), the United States Pharmacopoeia (www.usp.org), and the Joint Commission on Accreditation of Healthcare Organizations (JCAHO) (www.jcaho.org). Additionally, the Institute for Safe Medication Practices (www.ismp.org) makes communication and education about medication errors a priority.

The strongest predictor of patient outcomes is the quality of the communications between and among **health care providers**. Recognizing, responding to, and in turn preventing medication errors requires more than using the five rights of drug administration (right patient, right drug, right dose, right route, and right time), but also the right reason, and right documentation. Forty percent of errors occur in healthy patients and range in severity from an error having no significant effect to one causing disability or death. All persons involved in drug therapies must be alert to the risk of errors, including the person prescribing the drug, the transcriber of the order, pharmacist, nurse, and ancillary personnel, to the patient and medication administration records. The majority of medication errors are preventable; thus, the nurse is the first and the last line of defense against a medication error. This means that the nurse has a great deal of responsibility to ensure patient safety by knowing as much as possible about drugs.

Half of all preventable medication errors begin with the health care provider's **orders**. Medication errors at this stage result from the sheer number of drugs on the market and similarity of drug names. The most hazardous situation occurs when medications from two different classes have **sound-alike or look-alike names**. An error of this type results in effects that are different from what was intended. Studies have shown that the most common medication errors involve antibiotics, anticoagulants, antidiabetic drugs, antineoplastic drugs, cardiovascular drugs, central nervous system drugs, and vaccines. The Institute for Safe Medication Practices (ISMP) recently reported mix-ups occuring between two drugs with sound-alike and look-alike names. For example, the antifibrinolytic medication Amicar (aminocaproic acid) used for hemostasis can be confused with Omacor (omega-3 fatty acids), which is used to lower triglycerides levels. This example illustrates why the nurse must consult with the prescriber if the medication to be administered is not logical for the patient's condition. When preparing for medication administration the nurse also needs to be familiar with and cross reference the generic name of each medication.

The ISMP also warns about the danger of confusing various extended-release forms of the same drug. They point out that the problem is likely to increase as drug manufacturers expand their product lines to include more forms of the same drug. ISMP cites the example of Wellbutrin, which is now available as Wellbutrin, Wellbutrin XL, and Wellbutrin SR. Other problem medications include Metadate ER and Metadate CD, Ritalin LA and Ritalin CD, and Depakote and Depakote ER to name a few. The ISMP cautions that these various extended release formulations are not interchangeable.

Mix-ups may also be linked to poor **handwriting** along with the sound-alike, look-alike names. For example, mistakenly giving Amaryl (glimepiride), an antidiabetic drug, to a nondiabetic patient with Alzheimer's disease who should have received Reminyl (galantamine hydrobromide) has caused serious adverse events, including severe hypoglycemia and two deaths. Three other factors contribute to the possible confusion with these two drugs: both drugs were available as tablets, both come in 4-mg dosage strengths, and they both have generic names that placed them in close proximity to each other in storage. To resolve the issue of poor handwriting, all medication orders should be typed or printed (not cursive) if computer entry is not available.

Another area of possible medication errors involves miscommunication during transmittal of verbal and telephone orders. **Verbal orders,** which are orders spoken aloud in person or by telephone, offer more room for error than written orders or orders sent electronically. The interpretation of what someone else says is inherently problematic because of different accents, dialects, and pronunciations. Background noise, interruptions, and unfamiliar terminology often compound the problem. Transcription from a scrap of paper to the chart introduces another opportunity for error.

Once received, verbal orders must be transcribed as a written order, which adds complexity and risk to the ordering process. The only true records of a verbal order are in the memories of those involved. When the nurse records a verbal order, the prescriber assumes it was understood correctly. No one except the prescriber, however, can verify that the message was heard correctly. If a nurse receives a verbal order and then calls the pharmacy, there is even more room for error. The pharmacist must rely on the accuracy of the nurse's written transcription of the order and the pronunciation when it is read to the pharmacist. Faxes, electronic mail, and point-of-care computerized prescriber order entry are reducing the need for verbal orders in nonemergent situations. However, it is very unlikely that they will be totally eliminated. Never use verbal orders as a routine method of order communication. For example, do not accept verbal orders when the prescriber is present and the patient's chart is available.

Prescribers must communicate verbal orders clearly and the receiver should always repeat the order to the prescriber to avoid misinterpretation. This step is absolutely essential and should become habit even if the receiver is confident that the order was correctly understood. As an extra check, either the prescriber or listener should spell unfamiliar drug names, saying "T as in Tom," "C as in Charlie," and so forth. Pronounce each numerical digit separately, saying for example, "one six" instead of "sixteen," to avoid confusion with "sixty."

Medication errors also occur from misinterpretation of **abbreviations.** The NCCMERP recommends, and JCAHO requires, that certain abbreviations be avoided all together or written out in full. The ISMP provides a list of abbreviations, symbols, and dose designations that are frequently misinterpreted and involved in harmful medication errors. The complete list of abbreviations can be found at the ISMP website. An example is using the abbreviations *U* and *IU,* where the *U* can be mistaken as the number *0,* particularly when the *U* is written too closely after the number. This misinterpretation can lead to a 10-fold overdose. And *IU* can be mistaken for *IV* or the number *10.* Instead of using *U* and *IU,* use the terms *unit* and *international unit.* And then there is *q.d.,* meaning every day, and *q.o.d.,* meaning every other day. The abbreviation *q.d.* can be mistaken as *q.i.d.,* especially if the period after the *q* or the tail of the *q* is misinterpreted as an *i.* Further, *q.o.d.* can be mistaken for *q.d.* or *q.i.d.* if the *o* is poorly written. Instead, write out *daily* or *every other day.*

There is also the confusion caused by medication doses that include decimal points. A trailing zero after a decimal point can make a *1.0-mg* dose look like a *10-mg* dose if the decimal point isn't seen. Similarly, *.5 mg* can look like *5 mg.* So avoid trailing zeros for doses expressed in whole numbers, and be sure to use a leading zero when the dose is less than a whole unit.

Most oral medications are available commercially in the dosage strengths commonly prescribed. However, on occasion the patient's exact dose is not available, so more than one tablet or just part of a tablet may be needed. Whereas using more than one tablet for a single dose is customary, **tablet splitting** has become more commonplace in the past 5 years for several reasons: (1) assorted tablet strengths often cost about the same; (2) patients unable to afford their medications receive a higher strength tablet with directions to take ½ tablet (or even ¼ tablet) per dose; (3) some health insurers deny payment for lower strength prescriptions of certain drugs, thus requiring patients to receive the higher strength tablet to split in half for each dose; (4) health care organizations may not purchase all available strengths of oral medications, thus, some of the drugs may require tablet splitting for patient-specific doses in the in-patient setting; and (6) patients may not be able to swallow whole tablets.

Medication administration records often have methods for flagging unusual doses. Nurses need to be alert to these warnings. The nurse must also be sure that a medication can be cut; use an accurate pill cutter, and clean the device before and after use to prevent cross contamination with other patient's medications.

 ## Points to Remember

- The strongest predictor of patient outcomes is the quality of communication between and among health care providers.

- There is great danger for serious errors when medications from two different classes have sound-alike or look-alike names.

- Read back verbal orders to the prescriber to clarify the information.

- Avoid using abbreviations.

- An existing order may not be corrected, altered, added to, or modified in any way. If a change is needed, the order must be rewritten.

- Research a drug if you are unfamiliar with it. Clarify orders if you cannot read them. Document timely and properly. If you are unsure of anything, ASK!!!

 ## For Your Viewing Pleasure

Now check out the video clip for Module 6 on your CD.

 ## Learning Activities

Abbreviations

The following medication orders are from real-life situations. First, analyze the order and circle the component(s) in question. Rewrite the order to make it a correct, properly written, legally defensible medication order.

1. Morphine 2-5 mg IV q10min PRN pain

2. Lantus insulin subcutaneously 25 U each morning and 10 U each evening

3. Levothyroxine .125 mg by mouth daily

4. Coumadin 5.0 mg daily

5. Menest 0.3 mg po QOD

Complete the Lines

Fill in the squares using terms associated with medication errors.

1. _ C _ _ _
2. (2) _ _ _ _ _ O _ _ _ _ _
3. (2) M _ _ _ _ _ _ _ _ _ _ _ _ _
4. _ _ _ M _ _ _ _ _
5. U _ _ _ _
6. N _ _ _ _
7. (2) _ _ _ _ _ _ _ _ _ _ _ I _ _
8. (2) C _ _ _ _ _ _ _ _ _ _ _
9. (3) _ _ _ -A _ _ _ _ _ _ _ _
10. (2) _ _ _ _ T-_ _ _ _ _ _ _
11. _ _ _ _ _ I _ _ _ _ _ _
12. (2) _ _ _ _ _ _ _ O _ _ _ _
13. (2)_ _ _ _ _ -_ _ _ _ _ N _
14. (3) S _ _ _ _ -_ _ _ _ _ _ _ _

 Test Your Knowledge

Directions: Circle the best response.

1. a. You have the following medication order: Celebrex 200 mg po daily for 10 days. You go to the medication room and find Cerebyx in the automated dispenser. What do you do next?

   1. Recheck the order
   2. Contact the pharmacy
   3. Contact the physician
   4. Check the drug handbook

   b. This event would be considered a:

   1. Nurse error
   2. Pharmacy error
   3. Physician error
   4. Transcription error

2. Most drug errors occur when the nurse:

   1. Is responsible for administering numerous drugs
   2. Is caring for too many patients
   3. Fails to follow routine procedures
   4. Is administering unfamiliar drugs

3. The strongest predictor of positive patient outcomes is/are:

   1. Use of the correct drug
   2. Communication among and between health care providers
   3. Correcting poor handwriting
   4. Avoiding the use of abbreviations

4. You work in a 12-bed rural hospital where stock bottles and multidose vials of medications are stored, rather than the unit-dose system with which you are familiar. Your neurotrauma patient has developed status epilepticus. You are given a verbal order for fosphenytoin 15 mg PE/kg. Your patient weighs 80 kg. You find phenytoin 300 mg capsules and 1200 mg PE fosphenytoin prefilled syringes. On a separate sheet of paper, identify the factors in this scenario that increase the risk for medication errors.

5. On that same piece of paper, explain the difference between a drug's mechanism of action and its effects.

6. Nursing measures to reduce the risk of medication errors include which of the following?

   1. The nurse should never question the order a board-certified health care provider has prescribed for a patient.
   2. There are many sound-alike and look-alike medication names that should always be double-checked because of the high risk for error.
   3. When questioning an order for a medication, always assume that the prescriber is correct.
   4. Always go with your "gut" level feeling, and if you think a drug route has been incorrectly prescribed, it is acceptable to use the oral route for administration.

Answer Key

Module 6
Medication Errors

LEARNING ACTIVITIES

Abbreviations

1. The abbreviation *q* is not a JCAHO acceptable abbreviation since it may be confused with *q.i.d.,* especially if the period after the *q* is misunderstood as an *i.* Correctly written, the order should be: Morphine 2-5 mg IV every 10 min PRN pain.

2. Units should be written out. *U* may be confused with the number *0* or *4,* causing a 10-fold overdose. Correctly written the order should read: Lantus insulin subcutaneously 25 *units* each morning and 10 *units* each evening.

3. A *0* should always precede a decimal point to avoid mistaking this dosage for 125 mg. Correctly written the order should read: levothyroxine *0.125* mg by mouth daily

4. The decimal point in this example could be missed, leading to a 10-fold dosage error. Correctly written it should be: Coumadin 5 mg daily.

5. If the *o* is poorly written, *q.o.d.* could be mistaken for *q.d.* or *q.i.d.* The order should be correctly written as: Menest 0.3 mg po *every other day.*

Complete the Lines

1. **C**—JCAHO
2. **O**—Verbal orders
3. **M**—Medication error
4. **M**—Assumption

5. **U**—Units
6. **N**—Nurse
7. **I**—Poor handwriting
8. **C**—Clarify orders
9. **A**—Look-alike names
10. **T**—Tablet-splitting
11. **I**—Abbreviations
12. **O**—Decimal points
13. **N**—Tablet-splitting
14. **S**—Sound-alike names

TEST YOUR KNOWLEDGE

1. a. 1
   b. 2
2. 3.
3. 2.
4. a. Can't use *po* in place of *IV*
   b. Drugs are different
   c. Doses are not equivalent for the two drugs
   d. Working in a 12-bed rural hospital
   e. Unfamiliar dosing system
   f. Unfamiliar drugs
   g. Fosphenytoin cannot be given po
   h. Phenytoin po should not be given when an IV route has been ordered
   i. Oral drugs should not be given to a seizing patient
5. *Mechanism of action* is how the drug works in the body. *Effect* is the patient's response to the drug action.
6. 2

Module | 7

Drug Therapy with Pediatric Patients

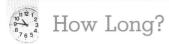

How Long?

Video: Approximately 3 minutes
Workbook: Approximately 60 minutes

Content Overview

Only a quarter of the drugs approved by the Food and Drug Administration (FDA) have specific indications in children and yet in the last decade, an estimated 12% of all prescriptions written in the United States were for children under age 9 years. Children differ from adults and from one another in regard to drug absorption, distribution, metabolism, and elimination. The pharmacokinetic and pharmacodynamic components of pediatric drug therapy are unique because of differences in body composition and the maturation of various organ systems. For the most part, OTC medications should not be taken by children under the age of 12 years, particularly aspirin because of its association with Reye's syndrome.

Children are not small adults. Drug therapy for children requires an understanding of the anatomic and physiologic differences between children and adults. The child is not only smaller in **height and weight** than an adult, but their proportions are also different. A child's weight increases about 20-fold between birth and adulthood, but height increases only 3.5-fold. The concept of body surface area (BSA) is important in pediatrics, because many physiologic functions are proportional to BSA.

Because drugs are water-soluble or fat-soluble at any given time, the percentage of **body fat** affects drug distribution. Body fat makes up approximately 16% of an infant's birth weight. Between the ages of 1 and 5 years, fat levels fall to 8% to 12%. The levels increase again by 18% to 20% of body weight at about age 10 years. Fatty tissue development reaches a peak at 9 months and then decreases again until about 6 years. In adolescence, subcutaneous fat tissue once again increases.

Body water is important as the medium in which solutes, including drugs are dissolved and as the medium in which all metabolic activities take place. Total body water throughout childhood is approximately 60% of body weight. During adolescence, the percentage of body water approaches that of an adult. Because of a child's greater proportion of body fluid, especially in the extracellular compartment, larger milligram per kilogram doses of certain drugs are required to achieve therapeutic drug levels.

ABSORPTION

As in the adult, drug absorption in infants and children depends on the route of administration, disintegration, dissociation, drug concentration, blood flow to the site, and absorptive surface area. Two factors affecting drug absorption from the GI tract are pH-dependent diffusion and gastric emptying time. Both processes are strikingly different in a premature infant compared with older children and adults. Age-related variables such as delayed gastric emptying time and irregular intestinal motility are examples of mechanisms that affect absorption. The rate of absorption also depends on the specific characteristics of the drug and the child.

Oral Route. Absorption of orally administered drugs is often delayed in neonates and young infants owing primarily to differences in pH and reduced gastric motility. Immediately after birth, gastric **pH** is low and therefore acidic drugs are less well absorbed. The pH reaches adult levels at about 2 years of age. Acidic drugs are less well absorbed. On the other hand, the absorption of acid-labile drugs (e.g., penicillin) may be enhanced.

Gastric emptying time is 6 to 8 hours in the neonate, but reaches the adult time of 2 hours by 6 to 8 months of age. Prolonged exposure of certain drugs to gastric contents increases the disintegration of unstable drugs and also delays drug entry into the lower GI tract, thereby delaying drug absorption and attainment of peak serum levels. Food can also interfere with drug therapy by altering the amount, type, and osmolality of gastrointestinal secretions, pH, transit time, and motility.

Parenteral Routes. The IV route of drug administration is commonly used in pediatrics. For some drugs, it is the only effective route. Intraosseous cannulation provides a reliable method for rapidly achieving venous access in emergencies, particularly in children younger than 6 years. The flat, anteromedial surface of the tibia, approximately 1 to 3 cm below the tibial tuberosity, is the preferred site. The marrow of long bones has a rich network of vessels that drain into a central venous canal, emissary veins, and ultimately into the central circulation. Medications and fluids gain entry to the central circulation within seconds by this route In general, the intraosseous route can safely be used to administer any drug or fluid formulated for IV use. This route is used temporarily until other venous access sites become available. IM drug absorption may be uncertain because of unpredictable blood flow, decreased muscle tone, lower muscle oxygenation, and vasomotor instability. Repeated injections in the child's few available muscle sites may cause tissue breakdown and less absorption of the drug. The absorption of drugs administered by the percutaneous route, however, is increased because of an underdeveloped epidermal barrier and greater permeability of the skin.

Topical Routes. The absorption rate of a topically administered drug is the same in a child as in an adult. However, more of the drug is absorbed in a child because of thinner skin and a greater BSA in relation to total body mass. Absorption of a topical drug is enhanced when occlusive dressings are used with the possibility of adverse reactions increased.

DISTRIBUTION

Many age-related differences in drug distribution occur during the first 10 to 12 months of life. The distribution of a drug in children is affected by the changing percentage of body fat, total body water content, total blood volume, and blood flow to target tissues. Drug distribution and equilibration rates may be faster in children than in adults. Therefore, a larger average dose per kilogram of body weight is needed to reach desired serum concentration levels. The higher the percentage of body water, the greater the dilution of water-soluble drugs. The result is reduced

serum concentration levels. As the percentage of body fat increases with age, so does the distribution of fat-soluble drugs. Therefore, the distribution of these drugs is more limited in children than in adults.

The immature liver of a newborn is unable to form **plasma proteins** (e.g., albumin), meaning their concentrations are 15% to 20% less than that of older children. Additionally, the albumin levels in neonates and infants result in lower binding capacity for certain drugs (e.g., penicillin) compared with the binding capacity of mature albumin. Thus, unbound drug levels can be high enough to produce side or toxic effects. To minimize the possibility of toxicity and to compensate for the shorter duration of drug action, it is often necessary to decrease the amount of the drug given, lengthen the time between doses, or both.

In contrast, adverse effects may occur when drugs, such as salicylates, penicillins, and sulfonamides, compete with endogenous substances (e.g., bilirubin) for the same protein binding sites. Competitive drug binding in the neonate increases the potential for adverse effects from increased concentrations of unbound, unconjugated bilirubin. Kernicterus (bilirubin encephalopathy) is a grave condition in which the basal ganglia and other areas of the brain and spinal cord are infiltrated with bilirubin. The greater permeability of the blood-brain barrier in children allows this to occur. Any drug that competes with bilirubin for protein binding sites or that inhibits the binding of bilirubin increases the risk. The signs of kernicterus are those of central nervous system depression or excitation, such as decreased activity, lethargy, irritability, loss of interest in feeding, seizures, and gastric or pulmonary hemorrhage.

METABOLISM

It is almost impossible to predict the effect of maturation on metabolism solely on the basis of age. Altered metabolic processes persist for approximately the first month of life but undergo a dramatic increase at about 6 months of age. During this time, however, the liver's **cytochrome P 450 enzyme system activity** is low, resulting in longer half-lives for some drugs (e.g., digoxin and acetaminophen). Dosages and choice of drug may be adjusted. In infants, for example, the antimicrobial drug chloramphenicol is inadequately metabolized reaching toxic levels; gray baby syndrome results. Chloramphenicol is associated with greater risk for mortality because of its longer half-life ($t_{1/2} = 26$ hr) compared to adults ($t_{1/2} = 4$ hr). Tachypnea, ashen-gray cyanosis, vomiting, loose green stools, progressive abdominal distention, vasomotor collapse, and possible death characterize this disorder. Discontinuing the drug as soon as symptoms appear may reverse the progression of symptoms.

Body temperature regulation is unstable in children, creating implications for drug action. When infants and toddlers develop an infection, the sudden high temperature increases the basal metabolic rate. For each degree centigrade rise in body temperature, the metabolic rate increases by approximately 12%. The higher metabolic rate reduces drug half-life and duration of therapeutic effects. Antipyretic effects of drugs are short-lived because of this phenomenon.

ELIMINATION

Most drugs are eliminated through three mechanisms: glomerular filtration, tubular secretion, and tubular reabsorption. **Glomerular filtration** is the most common mechanism. The glomerular filtration rate in infants is 30% to 50% of that in adults. Therefore, the half-life of drugs eliminated through the kidneys is approximately 50% longer than in adults. Additionally, during the first 6 months of life, an infant has a small number of renal tubular cells, a shorter tubular length, and a lower tubular blood flow resulting in reduced secretory capacity. Renal function reaches that of an adult at about 6 months of age. Drug dosages that depend on the kidneys for elimination must be adjusted to avoid toxicity from drug accumulation.

Drug elimination is also affected by **urinary pH**, because some drugs are more readily eliminated in acid urine and others require more basic urine. An infant's kidneys are less able to excrete hydrogen ions and reabsorb bicarbonate. As a result, the infant's urine is slightly less acidic than an adult's.

PHARMACODYNAMIC CONSIDERATIONS

Drugs produce the same mechanism of action in all individuals, including children. The patient's response to a drug, however, varies based on the maturity of the target organ and the maturity of the specific drug receptor. This area of pharmacology is receiving more attention as less invasive methods are developed to help identify the pharmacogenetics of individuals.

 Points to Remember

- Factors affecting the absorption of drugs from the GI tract include pH-dependent diffusion and gastric emptying time.

- The IV route of drug administration is commonly used in pediatrics.

- The higher the percentage of body water, the greater the dilution of water-soluble drugs, which results in reduced serum concentration levels.

- Inadequate albumin levels in neonates and infants results in lower binding capacity when compared with the binding capacity of mature albumin; unbound drug levels can be high enough to produce side effects or toxicity.

- Competitive drug binding in the neonate increases the potential for adverse effects from increased concentrations of unbound, unconjugated bilirubin.

- The liver's cytochrome P_{450} enzyme system activity is low, which results in longer half-lives for some drugs.

- The half-life of drugs eliminated through the kidneys in a neonate and infant during the first 6 months of life is approximately 50% longer than in adults.

- The patient's response to a drug's mechanism of action varies based on the maturity of the target organ and the maturity of the specific drug receptor.

 For Your Viewing Pleasure

Now check out the video clip for Module 7 on your CD.

 Learning Activities

Table Completion

Complete the table on the next page by identifying the nursing implications of drug therapies as they relate to the lifespan changes of infants and children.

Pharmacokinetic Phase	Developmental Changes	Implications
Absorption	1. Longer gastric emptying time	1.
	2. High gastric pH	2.
Distribution	1. Increased percentage of body fat	1.
	2. Decreased serum albumin levels	2.
Metabolism	1. Metabolic activity immature	1.
	2. Reduced microsomal enzymes	2.
Elimination	1. Reduced renal blood flow	1.
	2. Altered excretory capacity	2.

Fill in the Blanks

1. Total body _____ throughout childhood is approximately 60% of body weight.

2. Such age-related variables as delayed _____ _____ and irregular _____ motility are examples of mechanisms that affect absorption in a child.

3. The immature liver of a newborn is unable to form _____ (e.g., albumin), meaning their concentrations are _____% to _____% less than that of older children.

4. The signs of _____ are those of central nervous system depression or excitation, such as decreased activity, lethargy, _____, loss of interest in _____, seizures, and gastric or pulmonary hemorrhage.

5. The liver's _____ _____ _____ _____ activity is low, which results in longer _____ for some drugs.

6. A child's higher _____ rate reduces drug _____ and duration of _____ effects.

7. The GFR in infants is _____% to _____% of that in adults. Therefore the _____ of drugs eliminated through the kidneys is approximately _____% longer than in adults.

8. Children are not young _____.

Anagrams

1. patrons bio

   _____

2. do it rubs it in

   _____

3. mom tie slab

   _____

4. initial nome

   _____

Test Your Knowledge

Directions: Circle the best response.

1. The nurse anticipates that because of changes of drug distribution and equilibration rates in a child, the dose of a drug needed per kilogram of body weight to reach a desired serum concentration will be:

   1. Smaller than that needed by an adult
   2. The same as that needed by an adult
   3. Larger than that needed by an adult
   4. Uncertain and cannot be determined

2. Knowing that the albumin in neonates and infants has a lower binding capacity for penicillin, the nurse would expect which of the following to minimize the risk of toxicity?

   1. Decrease the dosage of drug ordered
   2. Increase the dosage of drug ordered
   3. Shorten the time interval between doses
   4. Make the time interval between doses irregular

3. A nurse considering the effect of renal function on drug elimination recalls that full renal function develops in infants by:

   1. 2-3 weeks of age
   2. 1-2 months of age
   3. 2-5 months of age
   4. 6-12 months of age

4. An infant is due for a dose of the antimicrobial drug chloramphenicol. The nurse notes in the record that the child has developed ashen-gray cyanosis, tachypnea, vomiting, and loose green stools. Which of the following actions would be most appropriate at this time?

   1. Administer the next dose as scheduled
   2. Administer the next dose one half hour later
   3. Give the next dose in twice the volume of fluid
   4. Withhold the dose and notify the prescriber

5. The nurse would assess which of the following single parameters as most useful in calculating drug dosages for a child?

   1. Age
   2. Body surface area
   3. Height
   4. Weight

Answer Key

Module 7
Drug Therapy with Pediatric Patients

LEARNING ACTIVITIES
Table Completion

Pharmacokinetic Phase	Developmental Changes	Implications
Absorption	1. Longer gastric emptying time	1. Prolonged exposure increases disintegration of unstable drugs and delays drug entry into the lower GI tract
	2. High gastric pH	2. Absorption of acid-labile drugs enhanced
Distribution	1. Increased percentage of body fat	1. Increased absorption of fat-soluble drugs
	2. Decreased serum albumin levels	2. More drug free in the circulation to act
Metabolism	1. Metabolic activity immature	1. Longer half-life of drug
	2. Reduced microsomal enzymes	2. Reduced metabolism and longer half-life of drug
Elimination	1. Reduced renal blood flow	1. Reduced elimination of drug
	2. Altered excretory capacity	2. Half-life 50% longer

Fill in the Blanks
1. Water
2. Gastric emptying time; intestinal
3. Plasma proteins; 15; 20
4. Kernicterus; irritability, feeding
5. Cytochrome P450 microsomal enzyme system; half-lives
6. Metabolic; half-life; therapeutic
7. 30; 50; half-life; 50
8. Adults

Anagrams
1. Absorption
2. Distribution
3. Metabolism
4. Elimination

TEST YOUR KNOWLEDGE
1. 3
2. 2
3. 4
4. 4
5. 2

Module | 8

Drug Therapy with Older Adults

How Long?

Video: Approximately 4 minutes
Workbook: Approximately 60 minutes

Content Overview

Persons over 65 years of age buy 35% of all prescription drugs and more than 40% of OTC drugs sold in the United States, at an annual cost exceeding $3 billion. The average older adult living at home uses 4 to 5 prescription drugs and 2 OTC drugs, refilling these drugs 12 to 17 times per year. Residents of extended care facilities average 7 to 8 prescriptions a year. The drugs most commonly prescribed for older adults include diuretics, potassium salts, histamine$_2$-antagonists, nitroglycerin, insulins, cardiac glycosides, beta-blockers, antianxiety drugs, and antihypertensives. The most common OTC drugs purchased by older adults are analgesics, antiinflammatory drugs, laxatives, and antacids.

Compounding the effect of physiologic aging on pharmacokinetics and pharmacodynamics is the presence of comorbid, chronic disease. The higher incidence of chronic diseases generally results in greater use of prescriptive and OTC drugs. **Polypharmacy** is the result of multiple disease processes, but also of the prescribing behaviors of health care providers and of poorly coordinated patient management. Polypharmacy results in a higher risk for adverse effects, drug interactions, extended hospital stays, and reduced compliance. Ironically, drug reactions that mimic medical-physical complaints are often treated with yet another drug. Further, many nurses assume that confused behavior is normal while it is commonly associated with drug reactions or interactions. The nurse should always determine the normal function of an older adult, even if they

are diagnosed with dementia (including Alzheimer's disease), and report any changes.

The rate of **side effects** is directly proportional to the number of drugs taken. Patients receiving two drugs have a 5.6% risk for an adverse drug interaction, whereas those receiving five drugs have a 50% risk. Patients receiving eight different drugs have a 100% chance for a drug interaction. Adverse drug reactions in older adults are responsible for more than 243,000 hospitalizations, 32,000 hip fractures, 160,000 changes in mental status, and 2 million cases of drug dependence annually. Although polypharmacy is significant in older adults, it is commonly overlooked as a factor in patient symptoms. In addition, excessive drug use by the older adult inadvertently creates an economically, psychologically, and physiologically costly cycle of events from which he or she may never recover.

One strategy that can be used to sort out drug interactions caused by polypharmacy is to have the patient bring in all of his or her drugs for review, including prescription and OTC drugs. The **"brown bag"** session allows the health care provider to check the appropriateness of medications for patients and their comorbid conditions. A brown bag session can also lead to the discovery of inappropriate drugs, duplication of drugs (e.g., brand name drug with a generic drug), older or expired drugs that should have been discontinued or thrown away, and supplements or OTC drugs that may not be listed in the patient's chart. Brown bag sessions can be included at health fairs or other community gatherings.

Although prescribing is in the hands of those with legal authority to do so, there are six **basic principles** that should be followed:

- Start low and go slow.

- Start one (drug), stop two.

- Do not use a drug if the adverse effects are worse than the disease.

- Use as few drugs as possible, choosing nondrug therapies when possible.
- Frequently assess the patient's response.
- Consider drug holidays from time to time.

CHANGES OF AGING

As we age, a variety of physiologic changes increase the older adult's sensitivity to drugs and drug-induced problems. However, note that chronological age is not necessarily related to physiologic age. With aging there is a gradual decline in many body systems, with some systems more affected than others. Indeed, the variations between people of the same age are so great that increased biologic variation is characteristic of this age group. Drug effects are different in older adults owing to either pharmacokinetic or pharmacodynamic factors.

Absorption

Comparatively speaking, older adults have less difficulty with drug absorption than with distribution, metabolism, or elimination. Drugs affecting gastric acidity, motility, or trypsin production (e.g., laxatives, antacids, anticholinergics, levodopa) alter the absorption of other drugs. Decreases in **gastric motility** and in the production of trypsin delay or impair drug absorption. Conditions such as increased **gastric pH** alter the absorption of weak acids and bases. For example, weak acids (e.g., barbiturates) are more ionized in the GI tract and less well absorbed. In contrast, weak bases are less ionized and better absorbed. As a result, older adults may not respond as quickly to an oral dose of a drug as people in other age groups.

Many indigestion problems seen in the older adult are related to increases in gastric pH and reduced amounts of hydrochloric acid (hypochlorhydria), pepsin, lipase, and pancreatic enzymes. The aging pancreas produces normal amounts of bicarbonate and amylase, but there is a decrease in lipase, resulting in subclinical abnormalities in fat absorption. Reduced fat absorption also reduces the absorption of fat-soluble vitamins, and there is faulty absorption of vitamin B_1, vitamin B_{12}, calcium, and iron.

In addition, the age-related decline in **cardiac output** results in a 40% to 50% reduction in perfusion of the GI tract. This is because blood flow to the area must be sacrificed to maintain coronary and cerebral blood flow. The result is delayed, less thorough, and less reliable removal of drugs and other substances from the intestinal lumen. Intestinal blood flow is decreased, which may reduce the absorption of substances actively transported from the intestinal lumen (e.g., some sugars, minerals, and vitamins). The intestinal mucosa atrophies, decreasing in surface area, and the intestinal musculature weakens. Peristalsis is slower, contributing to constipation.

Distribution

Alterations in circulation and changes in body composition affect drug distribution and equilibration rates. The changes occur because aging alters many of the factors that influence protein binding, volume of distribution, the amount of body fat present, and regional perfusion patterns.

Body weight decreases, especially in those older than 75 years, but the ratio of fat to lean body mass is usually greater. Adipose tissue levels increase from 18% to 30% in men and from 35% to 48% in women. The enlarged fat compartment increases the distribution of lipid-soluble drugs. In other words, changes in adipose tissue raise tissue concentrations and the duration of drug action while lowering plasma concentrations. For example, a highly fat-soluble drug (e.g., diazepam) has greater distribution that leads to an extended half-life.

The decline in total body water with age means that highly water-soluble drugs will have a smaller area of distribution. For example, drugs like gentamicin have elevated plasma concentrations in the older adult. Because drugs in this class are almost exclusively eliminated by the kidneys and renal function falls with age, the end result can be a dangerous accumulation of drug.

Reduced **plasma protein** (albumin) levels result in higher concentrations of unbound drug. The effect of this change is not always predictable. As the amount of unbound drug rises, the amount of drug available for producing an effect increases but so does the amount of drug available for biotransformation and excretion. For example, a highly protein-bound drug (e.g., phenytoin) undergoes greater metabolism, which decreases serum drug levels and therapeutic effects. In contrast, another highly protein-bound drug, such as warfarin, an anticoagulant, will produce greater effects in patients with low serum albumin levels.

Other factors altering drug distribution in the older adult include poor nutrition, extremes of body weight, electrolyte and mineral imbalances, inactivity, and prolonged bedrest.

Metabolism

Although the liver remains functional in the older adult, the ability to metabolize drugs declines. A person who lives to be 100 years old will have a 50%

reduction in liver mass, with the greatest decrease occurring between the ages of 60 and 70 years. Drug metabolism in the liver depends on two processes, **hepatic blood flow,** and **cytochrome P450** microsomal enzyme system activity. With aging, blood flow to the liver is reduced so that less drug is delivered to the liver. The reduced blood flow and lower enzyme activity can be particularly significant with drugs for which metabolic rates depend on hepatic blood flow (e.g., propranolol).

Although no significant effects have been reported, the smaller size and reduced function of the liver interferes with the formation of prothrombin, albumin, and vitamins A and D. Conditions such as dehydration, hyperthermia, immobility, and liver disease diminish the metabolism of drugs. As a consequence, drugs may accumulate to toxic levels. Also, the extended half-life of many drugs warrants close monitoring of clearance in older patients. Such drugs as morphine, meperidine, propoxyphene, propranolol, lidocaine, phenylbutazone, warfarin, amobarbital, and benzodiazepines have extended half-lives.

Elimination

With aging, the number of functional nephrons falls by as much as 64% and the **glomerular filtration** rate by 46%. The normal decline in glomerular filtration is not reflected in the serum creatinine, because of the comparable loss in muscle mass, which lowers the production of creatinine. This means that an older patient may not have higher serum creatinine levels until the dysfunction is severe. The change is accompanied by a similar decrease in renal blood flow. Tubular secretory mechanisms and the ability to concentrate urine are diminished. In addition, cardiovascular disease, dehydration, and kidney disease commonly impair renal functioning. Thus the half-life of a drug may be increased by as much as 40%. Because drugs remain in the body longer, the risk of adverse effects increases.

Points to Remember

- The goal of drug therapy in the older adult is to maintain health status using the fewest drugs possible.

- Increased adipose tissue of the older adult raises tissue concentrations and the duration of drug action but lowers plasma concentrations of the drug.

- As the amount of unbound drug rises, the amount of drug available to produce an effect increases, but so does the amount of drug available for metabolism and elimination.

- The half-life of a drug may be increased by as much as 40% owing to declining renal function, cardiovascular disease, dehydration, and kidney disease.

- Ideally, drug regimens are kept simple with the least frequent administration schedule used.

- Drug holidays reduce the likelihood that drugs will accumulate to toxic levels in the blood stream, increase mental alertness (in some cases), and provide a cost savings.

For Your Viewing Pleasure

Now check out the video clip for Module 8 on your CD.

Learning Activities

Fill in the Blanks

1. The drugs most commonly prescribed for older adults include _____, _____, _____, _____, _____, _____, _____, _____, _____.

2. _____ is not only the result of multiple disease processes, but also of the prescribing behaviors of health care providers and of poorly coordinated patient management.

3. The rate of _____ _____ is directly proportional to the number of drugs taken.

4. One strategy that can be used to sort out drug interactions caused by polypharmacy is to have the patient bring in _____ of his or her _____ and _____ for review.

5. _____ age is not necessarily related to physiologic age.

6. Decreases in _____ _____ and in the production of trypsin delay or impair drug absorption.

7. The age-related decline in _____ _____ results in a _____% to _____% reduction in

perfusion of the _____ tract resulting in _____, less thorough, and less reliable removal of drugs and other substances from the intestinal lumen.

8. The decline in total body water with age means that highly _____-soluble drugs will have a smaller area of distribution.

9. Reduced serum albumin levels result in _____ concentrations of unbound drug.

10. Drug metabolism in the liver depends on two processes, _____ _____ _____ and _____ activity.

11. With aging, the number of functional _____ falls by as much as 64% and the _____ _____ rate by 46%, resulting in _____ elimination of drug.

12. The top two principles of prescribing or administering drugs to the older adult are: _____ and

_____

Crossword Puzzle

Across

2. Alters the absorption of weak acids and bases

6. The result of multiple disease processes

8. To inform health care providers

9. Act as carriers for drug molecules

Down

1. Heart rate times the stroke volume

2. This function falls by as much as 64%

3. There are 6 of these

4. Drug metabolism depends on this

5. First principle in prescribing for older adults

7. Proportional to the number of drugs taken

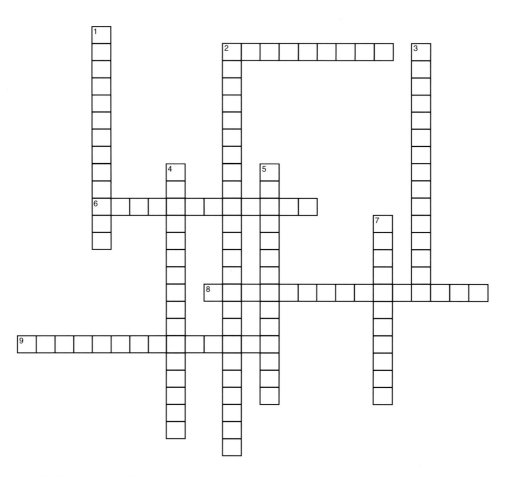

True or False

If the answer is false, correct the statement to make it true.

1. _____ Start one (drug), stop two.

2. _____ It is acceptable in some cases to use a drug when the adverse effects are worse than the disease.

3. _____ Chronological age is not necessarily related to physiologic age.

4. _____ A brown bag session is held so the patient and health care provider can get to know each other better.

5. _____ As the amount of unbound drug rises, the amount of drug available to produce an effect increases, but so does the amount of drug available for metabolism and elimination.

6. _____ Polypharmacy results in a higher risk of adverse effects, drug interactions, extended hospital stays, and reduced compliance.

Test Your Knowledge

Directions: Circle the best response.

1. The nurse caring for an older adult anticipates that which of the following states enhance drug absorption from the GI tract?

   1. Dehydration

   2. Hypotension

   3. Hypothermia

   4. Physical activity

2. An older adult is receiving the highly protein-bound drug phenytoin (Dilantin). Because of the effects of aging on blood components, the nurse understands that this drug will undergo:

   1. Greater metabolism, requiring smaller amounts of drug

   2. Greater metabolism, requiring greater amounts of drug

   3. Reduced metabolism, requiring smaller amounts of drug

   4. Reduced metabolism, requiring greater amounts of drug

3. The changes occurring in the kidneys of older adults have which of the following implications for the nurse who is assessing drug responses in this patient?

   1. Drug half-life is lengthened

   2. Drug half-life is shortened

   3. Drug elimination is faster

   4. Toxic drug levels are less likely to occur

4. The problem of polypharmacy in the older adult is less likely to occur when:

   1. The patient has several health care problems

   2. The patient uses large numbers of OTC drugs only

   3. There is poorly coordinated patient management

   4. There are a limited number of health care providers

5. Which of the following drug classifications are LEAST likely to place the older adult at risk for adverse effects and/or toxicity? Pick all that apply.

   1. Antianxiety drugs

   2. Antihypertensives

   3. Beta-blockers

   4. Cardiac glycosides

   5. Diuretics

   6. Histamine$_2$-antagonists

   7. Insulins

   8. Nitroglycerin

   9. Potassium salts

Answer Key

Module 8
Drug Therapy with Older Adults

LEARNING ACTIVITIES
Fill in the Blanks

1. Diuretics, potassium salts, histamine$_2$-antagonists, nitroglycerin, insulin, cardiac glycosides, beta-blockers, antianxiety drugs, and antihypertensives
2. Polypharmacy
3. Side effects
4. All; prescription drugs; OTC drugs
5. Chronological
6. Gastric motility
7. Cardiac output; 40; 50; GI; delayed
8. Water
9. Higher
10. Hepatic blood flow; cytochrome P$_{450}$ microsomal enzyme
11. Nephrons; glomerular filtration; reduced
12. Start low and go slow; start one (drug), stop two

Crossword Puzzle

Across
2. Gastric pH
6. Polypharmacy
8. Brown bag session
9. Plasma proteins

Down
1. Cardiac output
2. Glomerular filtration rate
3. Basic principles

4. Hepatic blood flow
5. Start low go slow
7. Side effects

True or False
1. True
2. False; It is NOT acceptable.
3. True
4. False; Check the appropriateness of medications for patients and their comorbid conditions.
5. True
6. True

TEST YOUR KNOWLEDGE

1. 4. Physical activity enhances circulation that in turn positively influences drug absorption. The other options hinder drug absorption.

2. 2. Phenytoin is highly protein bound, undergoes greater metabolism because of reduced albumin levels, which increases the amount of circulating drug. Since more drug is metabolized, the serum drug levels and therapeutic effects decline, requiring higher doses of the drug to maintain therapeutic effects.

3. 1. Renal blood flow, glomerular filtration, and the number of functional nephrons all decrease in older adults. This causes drugs to be eliminated more slowly, effectively lengthening their half-life and increasing the risk of toxic drug levels.

4. 1. The problem of polypharmacy in the older adult can be minimized when the actual number of health care problems is low, when there are few drugs being taken (either prescription or OTC), when there are limited numbers of care providers, and when care is well-coordinated among providers.

5. All of the drugs place the patient at potential risk for adverse effects.

Module | 9

Drug Therapy with Pregnant and Lactating Patients

How Long?

Video: Approximately 5 minutes
Workbook: Approximately 60 minutes

Content Overview

Medication use in pregnancy is common. On average, 50% to 80% of all pregnant women use at least one drug during their pregnancy, and many take more than one drug. Occasionally, drugs are used simply on an as-needed basis to treat pregnancy-related discomforts, such as nausea, headache, or constipation. However, some pregnant women need to take drugs throughout their pregnancy for chronic medical conditions such as diabetes, hypertension, or asthma. Women may need antibiotics or other drugs for the occasional infection that may appear during pregnancy.

The normal physiologic changes of pregnancy are related to hormonal changes, growth of the fetus, and the mother's physical adaptation to the changes that are taking place within her body. To understand how pregnancy influences drug therapy, it is important to understand the changes that occur in the mother and fetus.

PHARMACOKINETIC CONSIDERATIONS

Absorption

Absorption of a drug given IM is increased because pregnancy increases tissue perfusion by inducing vasodilation. The absorption of orally administered drugs is influenced by gastric acidity, the presence of bile acids, mucus, and intestinal transit time. Slow **gastric emptying** and prolonged **intestinal transit time** induced by pregnancy delays the appearance of orally administered drugs in the plasma, but also may enhance the absorption of lipid-soluble drugs. Gastric motility and tone are decreased because of the smooth muscle relaxation effects of progesterone. These changes in turn result in delayed gastric emptying, prolonged drug absorption, and lower peak drug concentrations. Reduced gastric acid secretion during the first trimester is thought to result from high levels of placental histaminase and other hormonal influences, particularly estrogen. During the third trimester, gastric acid secretion increases. Reduced GI tone also leads to prolonged intestinal transit time, especially during the second and third trimesters.

In addition, **pH** changes associated with heartburn and morning sickness, or the treatment of these symptoms with antacids, affects absorption of some orally administered drugs. Reduced gastric acidity slows the absorption of weakly acidic drugs (e.g., aspirin) but speeds the absorption of weakly basic drugs (e.g., opioids).

During pregnancy **total body water** increases by 7 to 9 liters in the absence of edema; 40% is distributed to maternal compartments and 60% is distributed to the amniotic fluid, placenta, and fetus. Given the increase in extracellular fluid during pregnancy it is not surprising that a considerable amount of sodium is retained. This change is accompanied by an increase in renal tubular reabsorption to prevent maternal sodium depletion. Increases in renin, aldosterone, deoxycorticosterone, human placental lactogen, and estrogen seem to enhance sodium levels.

Normally, the blood pressure does not rise despite increases in cardiac output and blood volume. Systolic pressures remain stable or fall slightly, whereas diastolic blood pressure drops more significantly. The changes begin in the first trimester and continue until the middle of pregnancy. At that time, there is a gradual return to prepregnancy blood pressure readings. Alterations in blood pressure are probably related to estrogen- and progestin-mediated decreases in systemic vascular resistance.

Distribution

Weight gain in pregnancy results from increases in body fat, total body water, and the products of conception. Distribution of fat-soluble drugs is influenced by these changes. For example, the higher percentage of **body fat** acts as a reservoir for fat-soluble drugs. Thus highly lipid soluble drugs tend to concentrate in tissues and show a volume of distribution much higher than the blood volume. Generally the impact of an increased volume of distribution reduces peak plasma drug concentrations, which decreases the amount of drug available to move to the site of action or to move to sites for elimination. The **half-life** of the drug tends to be prolonged by these mechanisms.

Drugs with low lipid solubility (i.e., water-soluble drugs) tend to be highly bound to plasma proteins. In pregnancy the level of plasma albumin, to which most acidic drugs are bound, falls. Basic drugs (e.g., propranolol) tend to bind to alpha-1-glycoproteins. Endogenous ligands, such as free fatty acids, compete with drugs for binding sites on both albumin and alpha-1-glycoproteins. Both of these changes increase the concentration of free drug in plasma and favor increased distribution as well as elimination of the drug. These changes are greatest for drugs with relatively low lipid solubility and high protein binding (e.g., benzodiazepines).

Metabolism

Drug metabolism is heightened by the effects of **progesterone.** Estrogen enhances the production of alpha- and beta-globulins, but the liver's production of albumin and total serum protein levels are reduced by 20%. As a result, liver clearance of drugs is increased, elimination is accelerated, and the half-life shortened. The hepatic microsomal enzyme system remains sensitive to inhibition as well as stimulation by certain drugs, just as in the nonpregnant state.

Contributing to lower serum albumin levels is the expansion of intravascular volume. The lowered serum albumin levels allow more unbound drug to be available for placental transfer, with the transfer occurring at lower serum drug concentrations than in a nonpregnant state. Albumin binding capacity is also decreased, mainly because of competition with endogenous factors, such as free fatty acids.

Drugs ordinarily expected to have a shorter half-life (e.g., antibiotics) have elevated concentrations during labor, when the hepatic clearance of drugs is thought to decrease. Metabolism also occurs in both the placenta and the fetal liver, although the contribution of the fetal-placental unit is thought to be very small.

Elimination

In the nonpregnant state, the kidneys receive 1000 to 1200 mL of blood per minute. Soon after conception the **glomerular filtration rate** (GFR) rises 40% to 50% as a result of increases in total body water. The GFR may peak at 150% of normal within 9 to 16 weeks. The rise in GFR increases elimination of amino acids, glucose, proteins, urea, uric acid, potassium, calcium, water-soluble vitamins, creatinine, and certain drugs. The dosage and frequency of administration may need to be altered. Pregnant women should also be evaluated for signs of toxicity as well as for evidence of subtherapeutic drug levels.

Drugs that are excreted unchanged (e.g., gentamicin, digoxin) are cleared in proportion to the creatinine clearance. Because blood flow through the liver is not appreciably changed in pregnancy, drugs depending solely on hepatic blood flow for clearance are removed from the body at the same rate as in the nonpregnant state.

FETAL-PLACENTAL CONSIDERATIONS

Absorption

The placenta has a high basal metabolic rate with energy needs supplied predominantly by oxygen and glucose. The placenta transports oxygen and nutrients to the fetus and clears urea, carbon dioxide, and other catabolites produced by the fetus. Gases and some molecules cross the placenta by simple diffusion. Transport depends on the concentration gradient, the size of the molecule, and the surface area available for transfer. The highest diffusion rate across placental membranes occurs with substances of low molecular weight, minimal electrical charge, and high lipid solubility.

Distribution

The effect of drugs on the fetus depends on whether the drug is distributed throughout the body or selectively. Many factors influence placental transfer of drugs, including physiochemical properties, molecular weight and configuration, ionization, lipid solubility, and protein binding.

Optimal **uterine-placental blood flow** is obtained with the patient in a right or left lateral recumbent or sitting position. Uterine blood flow is impeded by standing or by lying in a supine position. Any maternal position that does not optimize uterine blood flow decreases the potential for fetal drug exposure.

The placenta is not an impermeable barrier. Drug transfer via the placenta is greatest late in pregnancy. As pregnancy progresses, chorionic villi become more numerous, providing a greater surface area across which diffusion between the maternal and fetal circulations can occur. Near term, the membrane separating maternal and fetal circulation thins considerably; the fetal capillary endothelium is separated from maternal circulation by a single layer of fetal chorionic tissue. Inflammation, hypoxia, vascular degeneration, or partial separation of the placenta affects drug transfer just as it affects transfer of oxygen and nutrients to the fetus. For example, a woman with diabetes tends to have a larger, thicker placenta, creating a greater distance for molecules to travel before arriving in fetal circulation.

Circulating plasma proteins are a reservoir for drugs. It is important to remember that only a free drug is able to cross the placenta into the fetal compartment and that many drugs bind to the same proteins. One drug therefore may displace another, resulting in a potentially dangerous increase in free drug concentration.

Blood flow through the umbilical cord is an important factor in the transfer of freely permeable drugs. Cord compression jeopardizes circulation and hence the delivery of oxygen to and removal of wastes from the fetus. Cord compression thus also affects the delivery of drugs to the fetus. Likewise uterine contractions impair placental blood flow and reduce the transfer of intravenous drugs to the fetal compartment when bolus administration of a drug coincides with a uterine contraction.

Metabolism

Metabolism by the fetus is mainly an inactivation process whereby the fetal liver, adrenal glands, and placenta carry out metabolic reactions. It is important to know that the metabolites and intermediate compounds from these processes may be harmful to the fetus.

Although the fetal liver contains the adult complement of enzymes, the activities of these enzymes at term are only about half those of an adult. The fetus must rely on maternal processes to clear drugs from fetal circulation.

Only unbound drugs in maternal circulation cross the placenta to reach the fetus. Therefore the protein-bound component of plasma drug concentration is often discounted. The fetus, however, also possesses the ability to store drugs through plasma protein binding. The protein content of fetal plasma increases with gestational age. Fetal albumin levels usually exceed maternal levels at time of delivery. The high levels of bound drug in the fetus promote placental drug transfer as free drug crosses the placenta to replace drug bound to fetal proteins. The bound component also increases the overall fetal dose after a brief administration of a drug, thereby prolonging fetal and, perhaps more importantly, neonatal effects of a drug given to the mother. Following birth the neonate is removed from the benefit of maternal metabolism and must rely on its own limited ability to metabolize and remove a drug from its circulation. Hence, drug action following birth may be prolonged and may have adverse neonatal consequences.

Elimination

The presence of drug-metabolizing enzymes in fetal liver supports the notion that the fetus is capable of eliminating drugs. Drug metabolites have been found in fetal serum, but because metabolites freely cross the placenta in both directions, it has been difficult to prove that they are of fetal origin.

A water-soluble drug crosses the placenta slowly to reach the fetus, but once there, it undergoes rapid excretion by the fetal kidneys. However, fetal urine voided into the amniotic cavity constitutes a substantial portion of the amniotic fluid. As the fetus goes through the normal process of swallowing amniotic fluid, it ingests the drug or its metabolites that have been eliminated in fetal urine. The result is more prolonged fetal drug exposure.

Lipid-soluble drugs diffuse back across placental membranes to the mother, who provides the major route of elimination. Metabolites formed by the fetal liver are probably excreted in bile and deposited in meconium.

PHARMACODYNAMIC CONSIDERATIONS

A **teratogen** is any compound capable of interfering with embryonic or fetal development. The type and amount of drug, rate of elimination, extent of distribution to fetal tissue, gestational age, and fetal receptor function all influence the likelihood of a teratogenic effect. To prove that a drug is a teratogen, three criteria must be met: (1) the drug must cause a characteristic set of malformations; (2) it must act only during a specific period during gestation; and (3) the incidence of malformations should increase with increasing dosage and duration of exposure. More importantly, drugs that fail to cause malformation in animals may later prove to be teratogenic in humans. Thus *a lack of teratogenicity in animals is not proof of safety in humans.*

The **FDA classification system** (i.e., A, B, C, D, and X) for systemic drug use in pregnancy is based on the level of known risk the drug presents to the fetus. Drugs falling into the A category have the least likelihood of causing harm, while drugs in the X category are strictly contraindicated during pregnancy.

The **timing of drug exposure** determines how the fetus is affected. The fetus is most vulnerable during the first trimester. From conception to day 14 after conception, there is little morphologic differentiation. Exposure to teratogens at this time generally has an all-or-nothing effect on the zygote: either the zygote is damaged so severely that it is aborted or there are no apparent effects. The greatest risk for malformations in the fetus is during the period of organogenesis (15 to 60 days after conception). After the first trimester, drugs do not cause gross structural abnormalities but can still have toxic effects or affect growth and development. Drug exposure at this time can lead to brain damage, deafness, growth retardation, malignancy, stillbirth, or death.

DRUGS AND LACTATION

More than 60% of newborns are breastfed, with approximately 95% of breastfeeding women taking at least one drug during the first week after delivery. Almost all drugs transfer into **breast milk** to some extent based on their protein binding, lipid solubility, and ionization. The infant almost always receives no benefit from this exposure and is considered to be an "innocent bystander." If drug concentrations in the breast milk rise high enough, a pharmacologic effect can occur in the infant, raising the question of possible harm.

Although no FDA categories exist for breast-feeding like the ones for drug use during pregnancy, some drugs are absolutely contraindicated during breast feeding. The Committee on Drugs of the American Academy of Pediatrics (AAP) publishes a list of drugs and chemicals that transfer to breast milk. The list identifies drugs that are absolutely contraindicated during breast-feeding, drugs that require temporary cessation of breast-feeding, drugs that should be used with caution during breast-feeding, and drugs that are usually compatible with breast-feeding. The goal is to minimize the risk of potentially harmful drug exposure to the breastfed infant.

 Points to Remember

- Maternal factors affecting drug response during pregnancy include reduced tone and motility of the gastrointestinal tract, altered secretion of hydrochloric acid, weight gain, rises in fluid volumes and blood pressure, higher production of plasma proteins, and greater competition for plasma protein binding sites.

- Pregnant women should be monitored for subtherapeutic levels as well as signs of drug toxicity throughout pregnancy whenever taking any drug.

- Fetal factors affecting drug response include the fetus's immature hepatic and renal systems, reduced plasma protein binding sites, umbilical blood flow, immature blood-brain barrier, a high proportion of water to body mass, and placental metabolism.

- During pregnancy, serum albumin levels are reduced, prompting an increase in the amount of unbound drug. Unbound drugs in the maternal plasma cross the placenta into the fetal compartment.

- Teratogenicity is influenced by the timing of use of the offending drug, the characteristics of the teratogen, the mechanism of action that triggers changes in developing cells, the dosage of the offending drug, and susceptibility of the individual fetus.

- When possible, drug therapy for a breastfeeding woman should be delayed until her infant is weaned or is not totally dependent on breast milk for its nutrition.

- Minimize drug exposure to mother and fetus by:
  ○ Clearly identifying the need for any drug used
  ○ Using the safest effective drug available while avoiding use of newer drugs
  ○ Avoiding sustained-release, long-acting drugs and those with long half-lives
  ○ Using the lowest effective dose possible for the shortest possible time
  ○ Using topical or local therapy whenever possible
  ○ Having the mother take the drug immediately after breastfeeding

For Your Viewing Pleasure

Now check out the video clip for Module 9 on your CD.

Learning Activities

Table Completion

Complete the following tables by identifying factors that can enhance versus inhibit drug transfer across fetal-placental membranes.

Drug Transfer Enhanced by:	Drug Transfer Inhibited by:
a.	a.
b.	b.
c.	c.
d.	d.
e.	e.

Fill in the Blanks: Drug Therapy and Changes of Pregnancy

Complete the following sentences using the most accurate and grammatically correct descriptive term from the list that follows.

Slow; Slows; Slowed; Slowing

Delay; Delays; Delayed; Delaying

Increase; Increases, Increased; Increasing

Enhance; Enhances; Enhanced; Enhancing

Prolong, Prolongs, Prolonged; Prolonging

Reduce; Reduces; Reduced; Reducing

Decrease; Decreased; Decreases; Decreasing

Most; Least

1. Generally, the impact of an _____ in the volume of distribution _____ peak plasma drug concentrations, which _____ the amount of drug available to move to the site of action or to move to sites for elimination. The half-life of the drug would tend to be _____ by the changes of pregnancy.

2. _____ gastric emptying and _____ intestinal transit time induced by pregnancy _____ the appearance of orally administered drugs in the plasma but also may _____ the absorption of lipid-soluble drugs.

3. _____ gastric acidity slows the absorption of weakly acidic drugs (e.g., aspirin) but speeds the absorption of weakly basic drugs (e.g., opioids).

4. Estrogen _____ the production of alpha- and beta-globulins, but the liver's production of albumin and total serum protein levels are _____ by 20%.

5. Given the _____ in extracellular fluid during pregnancy, it is not surprising that a considerable amount of sodium is retained. This change is accompanied by an _____ in renal tubular reabsorption to prevent maternal sodium depletion.

6. Soon after conception the glomerular filtration rate _____ 40% to 50% as a result of _____ in total body water.

7. A water-soluble drug crosses the placenta _____ to reach the fetus, but once there, it undergoes rapid excretion by the fetal kidneys.

8. The timing of drug exposure determines how the fetus is affected. The fetus is _____ vulnerable during the first trimester.

Test Your Knowledge

Directions: Circle the best response.

1. A health care provider anticipates that the reduced gastric motility that occurs with pregnancy will have which of the following effects on pharmacokinetics?

   1. Delayed drug absorption

   2. Diminished drug metabolism

   3. Reduced renal elimination

   4. Unchanged drug distribution

2. Which of the following changes occuring during pregnancy is taken into account by the health care provider when prescribing drug therapy for a woman of 10 weeks gestation?

   1. Decreased renal blood flow and glomerular filtration rate

   2. Increased peripheral vascular resistance

   3. Increased gastric acid secretion

   4. Increased cardiac output

3. A health care provider would be most concerned about heightened drug transfer via the placenta if the patient was how far along in the pregnancy?

   1. 8 weeks

   2. 18 weeks

   3. 24 weeks

   4. 36 weeks

4. The greatest metabolism of drugs that cross the placenta and affect the fetus is accomplished by the:

   1. Fetal liver

   2. Maternal organs

   3. Placenta

   4. Umbilical cord

5. A patient who is breast feeding must take a prescribed drug once daily. The health care provider instructs the patient to take her daily dose just:

   1. after nursing the infant

   2. after the infant's longest sleep period

   3. before nursing the infant

   4. before the infant's longest sleep period

Answer Key

Module 9
Drug Therapy with Pregnant and Lactating Patients

LEARNING ACTIVITIES

Table Completion

Drug Transfer Enhanced by:	Drug Transfer Inhibited by:
a. Lipid solubility	a. Increased diffusion distance
b. Nonionized drugs	b. High molecular charge
c. Molecular weight less than 600	c. High molecular weight
d. Lack of significant protein binding	d. Drug bound to plasma proteins
e. Increased placental blood flow	e. Decreased placental blood flow

Fill in the Blanks: Drug Therapy and Changes of Pregnancy
1. Increased; reduces; decreases; prolonged
2. Slow; prolonged; delays; enhance
3. Reduced
4. Enhances; reduced
5. Increased; increase
6. Increases; increases
7. Slowly
8. Most

TEST YOUR KNOWLEDGE
1. 1
2. 4
3. 4
4. 2
5. 4

Module 10

It's All About the Patient

How Long?

Video: Approximately 4 minutes
Workbook: Approximately 60 minutes

Content Overview

Despite our best efforts, how good a job we do as health care providers, what and how much we know about drugs and therapeutics, and how attentive we are in providing the best patient education, it is often how the individual patient acts in his or her daily life that truly governs the success—or failure—of drug therapy. The purpose of **collaboration** among health care providers and patients is to enhance **quality of care** and improve patient outcomes. However, without an understanding of the patient's health belief practices, treatment objectives often fail.

HEALTH BELIEF PRACTICES

Health beliefs and practices are an integral part of every culture and society. The perspective of the individual is a major factor in how health and illness are defined in that community. Health beliefs reflect what is considered to be a healthy state, and what can be gained with intervention by a health care provider. For example, a patient who does not perceive dizziness and early morning occipital headaches as abnormal is unlikely to seek attention for the underlying cause, which is likely hypertension.

Illness is culturally defined. What is diagnosed as illness in one society may be viewed as a normal phenomenon in another. Further, within a single society, there may be a lack of consensus as to what signs and symptoms constitute illness. For some

persons, the term *normal* is not a statistical concept but a personal judgment. In other words, in a group of people with the same symptoms, some would seek medical care, whereas others would ignore the symptoms, failing to associate them with illness. Heavy reliance on signs and symptoms is one of the primary problems with the medical model of illness. Except for gross abnormalities, manifestations that differentiate normal from abnormal are vague. The challenge is to determine at what point a change in body structure and function becomes a sign or symptom of disease that requires drug therapy.

Cultural dimensions of the patient are also a vital consideration because a rich variety of cultural and ethnic backgrounds has resulted in a wealth of folk practices. Each of the five major ethnic subgroups in American society (i.e., White Americans, African Americans, Hispanic Americans, Asian Americans, and Native Americans) have culturally diverse health beliefs and practices that influence health and illness. The science of **ethnopharmacology** is attempting to bridge the gap between traditional use of medicinal plants and their role in health care today. The many factors that influence ethnopharmacologic practices are inherent in cultural beliefs about the causes of illness.

Ethnopharmacologic practices view the individual as a composite of psycho-socio-cultural-spiritual and physiologic forces that interact with the internal and external environments. This belief is in contrast to Western medicine, in which diagnosis of disease is made by categorizing pathophysiologic deviations in body systems. An exploration of folk beliefs and practices may reveal many cross-cultural similarities and, as such, may help explain epidemiologic differences in morbidity. The differences may also be indicative of the culture-specific significance placed on certain disease-related problems. Further, societal differences in health and illness-related practices influence both the degree to which a patient is aware of body symptoms and the decision to act on those symptoms. The relief of symptoms, or lack thereof, is not a reliable way to determine whether patient complaints are somatic or psychogenic in origin. In most cases, drugs work best when the patient has a positive outlook, takes the drug according to directions, and complies with recommended health-promoting dietary or lifestyle modifications.

Because of the increasing interest in self-care and the trend toward OTC or nonprescription drug use, the health care provider must understand factors that influence a patient's treatment choices. Inherent in this understanding is knowledge of the patient's environment, dietary practices, sleeping patterns, and activity levels. Health-illness beliefs and practices, past experiences with the health care system, educational level, religious beliefs, language barriers, support systems, and financial resources should also be considered.

HEALTH-ILLNESS BELIEFS AND PRACTICES

A patient's health-illness beliefs and practices and use of the health care system affect the patient's adherence to a drug regimen. When confronted with symptoms perceived to be minor or easily controlled, patients often seek self-care remedies or OTC drugs before seeking care from a health care provider. It is only when these attempts do not relieve symptoms, or the problem worsens that patients seek care from a health care provider. With continued emphasis on individual responsibility for health, the importance of self-care and self-treatment continues to increase. Individuals with the greatest trust in contemporary health care practices and technologies are least likely to purchase OTC drugs or to use questionably efficacious products on their own.

Self-treatment is not limited to OTC drugs. Non-Western traditional folk and cultural practices and beliefs are mysterious by Western standards. A patient's use of home remedies and self-treatment strategies is important to note. The health care provider practicing in the home or community setting is in a unique position to acquire information about health and illness practices that may be unavailable to providers in clinics or inpatient or extended care settings. Some of the most common practices are reviewed here.

Dietary Practices

A working knowledge of the patient's dietary practices is essential to evaluate adherence to drug therapy as well as to evaluate the risk of drug-food interactions. Drug-food interactions are not well understood, but such interactions can have dramatic

effects on the patient. For example, large amounts of leafy green vegetables eaten while taking the anti-coagulant, warfarin, can result in bleeding. Less dramatic reactions involve the absorption of drugs related to the timing of food intake. Drugs may also alter nutrient absorption, which over time, can lead to vitamin and mineral deficiencies. The health care provider should assess the patient's nutritional status before starting drug therapy and periodically thereafter to determine the need for dietary or vitamin supplements.

White Americans

White, non-Hispanic Americans define health and illness in many ways. Health is the ability to carry out activities of daily living, a state of physical and emotional well-being, or freedom from illness. Conversely, illness is often defined as an inability to carry out activities of daily living, the presence of disease symptoms and pain, and the malfunction of body organs. Examples of etiologies of illness are the breaking of religious rules, exposure to causative agents, punishment from God, drafts, climatic changes, and abuse of the body.

Seventy-seven percent of White American consumers regularly self-treat, with approximately 40% of the U.S. population using at least one OTC drug in any 48-hour period. Eighty percent of self-limiting illnesses and health problems can be treated with OTC drugs. Sixty-nine percent wait to see if the problem goes away on its own, and 6 in 10 Americans say they are now more likely to treat their own health conditions than they were in the previous years and are generally confident in the health care decisions they make. Forty-three percent consult a health care provider, 38% take a prescription drug, and 26% are taking dietary supplements.

African Americans

Sixty-four percent of African Americans report an increase in self-care compared to years past. This compares to 59% for all Americans. Additionally, African Americans are more likely to embrace the communal aspect of health care. Seventy percent of African Americans say they feel responsible to help friends and family make health decisions. This compares with 63% of all Americans.

The African and Caribbean cultures have influenced the health care beliefs and practices held by African Americans. This population describes health as the harmony of the body, mind, and spirit. Illness is viewed as a state of disharmony that results from natural causes or divine punishment. Survival depends on restoring and maintaining a balance of harmony with nature.

The health care practices are derived from a fundamental belief in the power of the supernatural. They include the use of herbs, spices, and roots. Health care advice may come from a "granny," who is a voodoo practitioner. The first line of treatment is often prayer and the laying-on of hands, although there are no universally accepted practices. The patients may turn to these practitioners as well as Western health care providers.

African Americans may use diverse home remedies. For example, cooked cornmeal and peach leaves are wrapped in cloth and placed over an inflamed area or wound infection. It is thought that bactericidal enzymes are produced through the process of fermentation. A raw potato poultice may be used to treat inflammation and wound infections. For open wounds, salt pork may be secured in a cloth and placed over the affected area. Epsom salts are familiar ingredients in many folk remedies. The extent to which folk medicine is used in the African-American population is not well understood. Discriminatory practices, unfair treatment, and difficult access to the health care system have caused many African Americans to distrust the Western traditional health care system and to seek other options for care.

Hispanic Americans

Hispanic cultural influences include European, Spanish, South American, and Indian folk beliefs. Eighty percent of the Hispanic American population consists of persons from Mexico, Cuba, and Puerto Rico. The remaining 20% are descendants of Central and South American peoples. The use of medicinal herbs and folk healers accompanied by religious rituals is representative of this group.

Thirty-nine percent of Hispanic Americans report fewer health problems compared to 48% of all Americans. Further, they are least likely to have visited a health care provider for any reason during the previous year. Hispanic Americans seek more options for treating common ailments and are less likely to have used supplements for general health compared to all Americans. Seventy-two percent of Hispanic-Americans say they feel responsible to help friends and family make health care decisions. This compares with 63% of the general public.

Many Hispanic Americans believe that health results from good luck, as a reward for good behavior, or as a reward from God. Health represents equilibrium in a universe where the forces of "hot" and "cold" must be balanced. Body fluids reflect this perspective. Blood is hot and wet, phlegm is cold and wet, yellow bile is hot and dry, and black bile is cold and dry.

The concept of hot and cold forces originated with the early Hippocratic theory of health and the four humors. Health exists when the four humors are balanced, and health is maintained by diet and other practices. Cold foods are to be avoided during menstruation and after childbirth. Examples of cold foods are chicken, honey, avocados, bananas, and lima beans. *Friadad del estomago,* a "cold stomach," is caused by eating too many cold foods. In contrast, a pregnant woman avoids "hot foods", such as chocolate, coffee, cornmeal, garlic, kidney beans, onions, and peas. For restoration of health, hot diseases require cold treatments, and cold diseases need hot treatments.

Illness is also caused by "dislocation of body parts" or supernatural forces outside the body, such as *mal de ojo,* or "evil eye." *Envidia,* envy, causes illness and bad luck. Many people of Hispanic background believe that to succeed is to fail; that is, when a person's success provokes the envy of friends and neighbors, misfortune or illness may follow.

Hispanic Americans use a variety of remedies to prevent or treat illness. Novena candles may be burned to ward off evil. *Jabon de la mano milagrosa* (soap of the miraculous hand) cleanses and protects a person. Amulets such as *milagros* are worn to protect from evil. The *mano negro* (Black Hand) amulet of Puerto Rico may be placed on a baby at birth to protect it from the "evil eye." In addition, manzanilla, an herb made into tea, is used to treat abdominal pain, uterine cramps, anxiety, and insomnia. The star-shaped seeds of anise are used to treat painful gases, upset stomach, colic, and anorexia and to increase breast milk. Several levels of practitioners, one of whom is the *curandero,* may carry out the folk system of medicine, incorporating herbs, spices, and the power of divine intervention.

Asian Americans

Asian Americans have emigrated from China, Hawaii, the Philippines, Korea, Japan, Laos, Cambodia, and Vietnam. The Asian American folk medicine practices evolved from China and the Far East and comprise complex and varying methodologies. Imbalance between *yin* (female, negative energy) and *yang* (male, positive energy) causes illness. Restoring the balance is the basis for most therapies, including acupuncture, herbal medicines, massage, tai chi, skin scrapings, and cupping. Instead of destroying the "germs" that cause illness, much of folk medicine practice focuses on self-restraint, corrective diets, and herbs to restore balance. The body is seen as a gift given by parents and forebears that must be cared for and maintained rather than as an individual's property. The primary role of the health care provider in ancient China was to safeguard the body and to prevent illness.

Traditional remedies used to prevent and treat ailments among Asian Americans include *jen shen lu jung wan.* This brown, thick liquid is used as a general tonic to support the body system and aid in digestion. *Tiger balm* is a salve used for temporary relief of minor aches and pains. *Huo li jian mei su* are small, brown, coated tablets taken twice a day to relieve fatigue, to counteract senility, and to maintain youth, health, and vigor. *White flower* is a liquid used to treat colds, influenza, headaches, and coughs. *Thousand-year eggs* are uncooked eggs that are covered with carbon and straw and stored in large vases for extended periods. They are eaten daily with rice for good health.

Ginseng root is the most widely known of the Chinese herbs. It has universal medicinal usage in "building the blood," especially after childbirth. Chinese legend has it that the more the root looks like a man, the more effective it is. Native to the United States, ginseng is used as a restorative tonic. It has scientifically-proven antioxidant, antitumor, and antiviral effects.

Because of the focus on prevention in Asian medicine, many patients combine Western treatment with folk remedies. Assessments by the health care provider would include a review of all current treatment regimens. They may use folk remedies rather than seeking medical treatment, with sometimes serious consequences.

Native Americans

There are approximately 170 distinct Native American tribes in the United States; each with various health care beliefs and values. Consequently, it is difficult to generalize cultural and health belief systems. Medicine, magic, and religion are closely bound beliefs for most Native American peoples. The concept of medicine extends beyond the treatment of illness to include life and death, and harmony with the universe. To stay healthy, one must maintain a positive, balanced, intimate spiritual relationship with nature and must treat the body and earth with respect.

Another interpretation of the Native American view of health is that the body is partitioned into halves, plus and minus. There are also positive and negative energy poles. Every person has the power to control the self, and with this energy, spiritual control (control of the body's energy) is derived. Health is then characterized as a harmony between the halves, or the energy poles. Illness is disharmony of the body, mind, and spirit.

The Navajo people view illness as the result of displeasing holy people, annoying the elements, disturbing plant and animal life, neglecting the celestial

bodies, misusing a sacred ceremony, or tampering with witches or witchcraft. Sweat lodges were used by many native people to purify and detoxify. The Hopi people associate illness with evil spirits and therefore strive to avoid or ward off these spirits. An eastern band Cherokee medicine man, Hawk Littlejohn, describes illness as the imbalance of the body, mind, or spirit caused by an excess in one domain and the neglect of the other. For example, a student who spends too much time studying (developing the mind) may neglect the body and spirit and is therefore susceptible to disharmony and illness.

To treat disharmony and illness, the Native American may wear a thunderbird amulet for protection and good luck. One may wear a mask to hide self from the devil or evil spirits. *Estafiate* are dried leaves made into a tea to treat stomach problems. A medicine man may burn sweet grass in a purification rite or create sand paintings in an elaborate diagnostic ceremony. The way the medicine man's hand moves while casting the sand indicates a specific illness. Correct treatment may then be prescribed. In some areas the medicine men work in consultation with health care providers in western health care systems.

Religious Beliefs

Religious practices and beliefs of the patient must be taken into account by the health care provider when prescribing drugs and treatments. The beliefs of some religious groups (e.g., Jehovah's Witnesses) prohibit the use of blood and blood products and support other therapies, such as faith healing and prayer. Christian Scientists believe in the power of prayer as a healer. An assessment of the patient's specific beliefs and practices is necessary to provide comprehensive and patient specific health care. The legal implications of the religious practices as they relate to the patient's health care must also be acknowledged.

Drug Use and Misuse

The health care provider needs to be aware of the possibility of drug misuse *or* drug abuse. The patient's drug history should include use of illicit drugs, alcohol, and nicotine, all of which can significantly influence the effects of other drugs. Though the patient may be hesitant to disclose such information, the health care provider may be the first to detect substance abuse.

Language Differences

The health care provider should consider the patient's health care beliefs and use of non-Western treatments when considering drug options and the patient's potential for adherence. As mentioned previously, ethnic groups often use folk remedies and folk healers because of unfamiliarity with, distrust, or dislike of the health care system. Differences in language impair access to health care and may further discourage use of the system. Differences in language may interfere with the health care provider's ability to accurately assess the concerns and symptoms and ability to educate the patient. The use of nonfamily interpreters may facilitate an accurate assessment of health care concerns and drug use or abuse.

Family Support Network

An assessment of the patient's family network support is an important component in understanding the patient. Family living arrangements, the number, ages, and relationships of people in the home, communication patterns, the roles of family members, the power and authority structure of the family, and the presence of a caregiver all affect patient care. To effectively treat the patient, the health care provider must gain the trust of the patient's family.

Education

Nearly 20% of the U.S. population is functionally illiterate. A subtle approach is necessary to assess a patient's ability to read and comprehend directions for prescribed and nonprescription drug therapy. Patients who are unable to read or comprehend are often ashamed of the deficit and try to compensate by indicating that they understand and will comply. By having the patient read a drug label and explain how the product is to be taken (e.g., times, before or after meals, amount) the health care provider can assess the patient's vocabulary, knowledge of the drug, and comprehension level. The patient's knowledge of the drug may also be assessed through questioning about drug action, adverse effects, and the disease process. The discussion must involve not only the use of the drug but how and why to read a label. When covering patient education issues, don't forget to consider the patient's ability to open medication bottles, particularly patients with arthritis, strokes, paralysis, or other limitations.

Economic Factors

The high cost of pharmaceuticals is a common reason for the patient's lack of adherence with drug therapy. An assessment of the socioeconomic level and the availability of health insurance may provide the health care provider with information that will assist in prescribing the most cost effective drugs for the patient. Assistance programs commonly require a financial needs assessment to determine eligibility. Interpretation of eligibility regulations often becomes the health care provider's responsibility. Many patients regard self-treatment as a more economical alternative, both in time and in money, and may try this approach rather than seeking care from a health care provider. Astute pharmacists help patients save money by offering less expensive generic drugs or educating the patient about similarities and differences between products.

Available transportation and pharmacy delivery services may help patients obtain needed drugs. Health care providers and pharmacists can furnish information about delivery services to the patient when the cost of transportation or the inability to drive may prevent access to a pharmacy. It is also possible to obtain pharmaceuticals by mail, through a variety of pharmacy plans and manufacturers. For example, many older adults purchase their drugs through at a reduced price through the American Association of Retired Persons (AARP).

Patient Education

Patient education is seen as vital to the successful outcome of drug therapy. By educating the patient about the drugs being taken, the health care provider can elicit the required level of participation. The void between a patient's knowledge level and what information is needed for adherence is referred to as a **learning deficit**. To reduce side effects, knowledge of the drug's possible side effects, the time when these effects are likely to occur (if any), and the early signs that a reaction is developing must be known.

A great amount of time can be spent in pharmacotherapeutic teaching-learning activities. Yet poor understanding of verbal instructions and written materials remains a major factor in failure to achieve treatment objectives. Patients vary greatly in their ability to hear, read, and translate verbal language and written instructions into a meaningful whole. Close attention should be given to the patient's reading and comprehension abilities. Adherence to therapy is best achieved when both verbal and written information is presented at the appropriate level of understanding.

Educating the patient requires that the health care provider apply basic principles of teaching and learning. The health care provider needs to assess the patient or acquire information about the patient, such as age, gender, culture or ethnic background, educational, and comprehension level—all of these factors can influence the method and effectiveness of teaching and learning activities. Physiologic factors such as vision or hearing deficits may require alterations in teaching strategies. The health care provider will be more successful in educating the patient when the amount and specific content is tailored to the patient's interest, knowledge base, motivational level, self-care requirements, literacy, and cognitive abilities. The health care provider must remember the key concept that learning and motivation are enhanced by positive reinforcement. Written materials may be helpful but should be appropriate for the patient's reading and comprehension abilities.

Evaluation of Outcomes

Methods available to assess the degree of patient adherence and self-satisfaction with the treatment regimen may include pill counts, the review of a drug diary, self-reports, direct observation, assessment of physiologic parameters, and input from other health care workers, family members, or friends. Combining several methods provides a more accurate assessment.

Satisfaction with the treatment regimen is an important consideration that is often ignored or skimmed over when evaluating drug effectiveness. However, patient satisfaction is closely tied to adherence. Dissatisfaction may lead to nonadherence and failure of an otherwise adequate drug regimen. Dissatisfaction can be prevented if therapy is designed around the patient's life-style, resources, preferences, and health care needs. Hence, patient and family involvement is a necessity.

Points to Remember

- The perspective of the individual is a major factor in how health and illness are defined in a community.

- Cultural dimensions of the patient are vital consideration in pharmacotherapeutics because the rich variety of patients' cultural and ethnic backgrounds has resulted in a wealth of folk practices.

- Satisfaction with the treatment regimen is often ignored or skimmed over when evaluating drug effectiveness.

- Educating the patient requires that the health care provider apply basic principles of teaching and learning.

For Your Viewing Pleasure

Now check out the video clip for Module 10 on your CD.

Learning Activities

Ethnopharmacology

Fill in the boxes to complete the words associated with ethnopharmacology. The numbers in parenthesis indicate the number of words.

1. _ _ _ _ _ _ E
2. _ _ T _ _ _ _ _ _ _ _
3. (2) H _ _ _ _ _ _ _ _ _ _
4. _ _ _ N _ _ _
5. _ _ _ _ _ _ _ O _
6. (2) _ _ _ _ _ P _ _ _ _ _ _
7. H _ _ _ _ _ _ _
8. _ _ _ _ A _ _ _ _ _ _ _ _ _
9. (2) _ _ _ _ _ _ _ R _ _ _ _
10. (2) _ _ _ _ _ M _ _ _ _ _ _
11. _ _ _ _ _ _ _ _ A _ _ _ _
12. C _ _ _ _ _ _ _ _ _ _ _ _
13. (3) _ _ _ O _ _ _ _ _ _ _ _
14. (3) _ _ _ L _ _ _ _ _ _ _
15. O _ _ _ _ _ _ _
16. (2) _ _ _ _ _ _ G _ _ _ _ _ _
17. (2) _ _ _ _ _ _ _ _ Y _ _ _ _ _ _

True or False

If the answer is false, correct the statement to make it true.

1. _____ The perspective of the health care provider is a major factor in how health and illness are defined in a community.

2. _____ The purpose of collaboration among health care providers and patients is to enhance quality of care and improve patient outcomes.

3. _____ Ethnopharmacology views the individual as a composite of psycho-socio-cultural-spiritual and physiologic forces that interact with the internal and external environments.

4. _____ A patient's health-illness beliefs and practices and use of the health care system do not affect the person's adherence with a drug regimen.

5. _____ The void between a patient's knowledge level and what information is needed for adherence is referred to as a teaching deficit.

Strategies for Improving Adherence

Possible causes for nonadherence with drug therapy are identified on the left in the table below. Identify two or three possible solutions to each.

Possible Reasons for Nonadherence	Possible Solution(s)
Inability to pay for prescribed drugs	1. 2. 3. 4.
Lack of transportation to obtain drugs	1. 2.
Forgetfulness	1. 2. 3. 4.
Confusion surrounding disease, multi-drug regimen, directions, or instructions	1. 2. 3. 4. 5. 6. 7.
Unable to tolerate adverse effects of drugs	1. 2. 3.
Interference with prescribed drug regimen because of use of self-treatment strategies	1. 2. 3.
Overdosing, underdosing, or misusing drug based on perception of need for the drug	1. 2. 3.
Expiration or refilling of prescription or supplies prior to follow-up appointment with health care provider	1.
Multiple comorbid conditions or fatigue	1. 2. 3. 4.

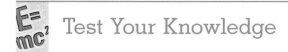 Test Your Knowledge

Directions: Circle the best response.

1. The health care provider questions a patient about the use of home remedies as part of an assessment of psychosocial considerations related to drug therapy. Data obtained as a result of this assessment would be most logically clustered or documented under which of the following categories?

   1. Environment
   2. Dietary practices
   3. Health-illness beliefs or practices
   4. Family support systems

2. Patients may have difficulty remembering to take prescribed drugs. The health care provider should try which of the following strategies first to help the patient adhere to their drug therapy?

   1. Have a community health care provider make a daily visit to administer the drugs.
   2. Perform pill counts every evening to check for missed doses.
   3. Schedule drug administration to coincide with meals or other routine activities.
   4. Use a drug diary to record all drug doses taken.

3. The purpose of collaboration among health care providers and patients is to enhance _____ _____ and improve patient outcomes.

4. Which of the following variables should be considered when planning a patient's drug therapy regimen? Caution: there may be more than one correct answer.

   1. Health-illness beliefs and practices
   2. Past experiences with the health care system
   3. Educational level
   4. Religious beliefs
   5. Language barriers
   6. Support systems
   7. Financial resources

5. Many Hispanic Americans believe that health represents equilibrium in a universe where the forces of "hot" and "cold" must be balanced. Body fluids reflect this perspective. Which body fluid is missing in the table below?

	Hot	Cold
Wet		Phlegm
Dry	Yellow bile	Black bile

Answer Key

Module 10
It's All About the Patient

LEARNING ACTIVITIES

Ethnopharmacology

1. Culture
2. Satisfaction
3. Health beliefs
4. Illness
5. Motivation
6. Health practices
7. Hispanics
8. Dissatisfaction
9. Asian American
10. Black Americans
11. Transportation
12. Collaboration
13. Lack of consensus
14. Ability to pay
15. Outcomes
16. Learning deficit
17. Culturally defined

True or False

1. False; individual
2. True
3. True
4. False; health care beliefs do influence health care practices
5. False; teaching deficit

Strategies for Improving Adherence to Drug Therapy

Possible Reasons for Nonadherence	Possible Solution(s)
Inability to pay for prescribed drugs	1. Consider cost of drugs when choosing therapy; use generic when possible 2. Minimize number of drugs prescribed; avoid polypharmacy 3. Use therapeutic alternatives when possible 4. Refer patient to appropriate agency for financial assistance
Lack of transportation to obtain drugs	1. Refer patient to appropriate agency for assistance 2. Explore pharmacy delivery or mail-away prescription services
Forgetfulness	1. Advise patient to bring all drugs (prescription and OTC) to each appointment 2. Choose a drug with fewest daily required doses 3. Use calendars, diaries, medication planners, or dosage containers 4. Review drug treatment regimens with family, friends, neighbors, home care personnel
Confusion surrounding disease, multi-drug regimen, directions, or instructions	1. Review risks and benefits of adding a drug 2. Explore non-drug therapies when appropriate 3. Review drugs added by other health care providers; communicate changes in therapy; provide a portable prescription record that can be taken to other physicians and pharmacists 4. Simplify drug regimen, directions, and instructions; use both generic and brand names on instructions 5. Make sure prescriptions are clearly labeled 6. Provide written as well as verbal instructions 7. Color code bottles; use large print materials as needed
Unable to tolerate adverse effects of drugs	1. Adhere to the principles: "start low and go slow", "start one, stop two" 2. Closely monitor patient condition; consider possibility that any new symptoms could represent adverse drug reactions or drug withdrawal symptoms 3. Consider changing to another drug, reducing dosage, or frequency of administration

Possible Reasons for Nonadherence	Possible Solution(s)
Interference with prescribed drug regimen because of use of self-treatment strategies	1. Reassess preferred treatment strategies 2. Educate patient 3. Provide large-print handouts to take home
Overdosing, underdosing, or misusing drug based on perception of need for the drug	1. Educate patient 2. Provide large-print handouts to take home 3. Closely monitor patient profile during regular visits
Expiration or refilling of prescription or supplies prior to follow-up appointment with health care provider	1. Closely monitor patient profile
Multiple comorbid conditions or fatigue	1. Schedule routine follow-up appointments to reevaluate patient condition 2. Choose one drug that treats two comorbid conditions when possible 3. Schedule regular blood tests to monitor patient response to diuretics, ACE inhibitors, antiseizure drugs, anticoagulants, antiarrhythmics, and digoxin 4. Stay informed about pharmaceutical innovations (novel new drugs, new diagnostics for predicting drug response, etc.) relevant to disease of older adults

TEST YOUR KNOWLEDGE

1. 3
2. 3
3. Quality of care
4. All are correct
5. Blood

Glossary

Abbreviations
Shortened forms or symbols for words that could potentially lead to medication errors as a result of misinterpretation.

Absorption
The movement of a drug from the administration site to the circulation (e.g., from the stomach to the circulation, from the muscle to the circulation). Absorption is needed for a drug to produce a pharmacologic action.

Active ingredients
Ingredients responsible for producing drug action. The major classes of active ingredients include alkaloids, glycosides, polypeptides, salts, and steroids.

Active transport
The movement of drug molecules against a concentration gradient using metabolic energy in the form of adenosine triphosphate (ATP).

Affinity
The degree to which a drug binds with a receptor.

Agonist
Any compound, either natural or synthetic, that stimulates specific drug receptors.

Antagonists
A drug that has an affinity for receptors, but which itself has no intrinsic activity; as long as the drug occupies the receptor site, other potential suitors are blocked from getting to that receptor.

Bioavailability
Term used to quantify the extent of drug absorption; the amount of drug actually available to the body to produce an effect at the receptor site.

Body fat
The amount of fat in the body; affects distribution of fat-soluble drugs.

Body water
Broad term for total body fluids; the medium in which solutes, including drugs, are dissolved.

Brand or trade name
The name a manufacturer assigns a drug, which is copyrighted by the pharmaceutical company and is legally on record for 20 years.

Breast milk
Milk made by the breast. All drugs transfer to breast milk to some extent based on their protein binding, lipid solubility, and ionization.

Brown bag session
A session that requires a patient to bring in all of his or her prescriptions and OTC drugs for review; the session allows the health care provider to check the appropriateness of medications for patients and their comorbid conditions.

Chemical name
Drug name based on the compound's precise chemical structure; name conforms to a specific set of international rules. These names are complex and therefore not practical for everyday use.

Clearance (CL)
The rate at which a substance is removed or cleared from the body by the kidneys and/or in renal dialysis. Clearance reflects the integrity of glomerular filtration.

Collaboration
The partnership between health care providers and patients to enhance the quality of care.

Creatinine clearance
In renal physiology, creatinine clearance (CrCL) is the volume of blood plasma that is cleared of creatinine per unit time. Clinically, creatinine clearance is a useful measure for estimating the glomerular filtration rate (GFR) of the kidneys.

Cytochrome P450 enzyme system
A general term referring to the wide variety of tissue enzymes (primarily in the liver) that play a significant role in drug metabolism.

Distribution
The delivery of drug molecules to the site of action; factors influencing the distribution of an absorbed drug include plasma protein binding, blood flow, tissue binding, and solubility.

Drug receptors
Any part of a cell that reacts with a drug, providing that each drug structurally conforms to the receptor site; proteins on cell membranes are the most important drug receptors.

Duration of action
The length of time a drug's concentration is sufficient to elicit a therapeutic response.

Efficacy
The degree to which a drug is able to produce maximal effects.

Elimination
The movement of a drug or its metabolites from the tissues back into the circulation and then to the organs of elimination.

Ethnopharmacology
The science that attempts to bridge the gap between traditional use of medicinal plants and their role in health care today.

FDA classification system
A classification system for systemic drug use in pregnancy based on the level of known risk the drug presents to the fetus; drugs are categorized as A, B, C, D, or X.

Formulations
The form a drug takes (e.g., creams, foams, gels, aerosols); designed to promote either local or systemic drug action or effects.

Gastric emptying time
The time it takes for the stomach to empty its contents.

Gastric motility
Movements of the stomach that aid in digestion; decreases in gastric motility delay or impair drug absorption.

Gastric pH
The acidity or alkalinity of the stomach; increased gastric pH alters the absorption of weak acids and bases.

Generic name
A drug name that is simpler than the chemical name and identifies or classifies the drug in scientific literature.

Glomerular filtration
The most common mechanism by which drugs are eliminated from the body; the kidneys use this method to rid the body of unchanged, unbound drug molecules and their metabolites.

Glomerular filtration rate (GFR)
The amount of ultrafiltrate formed per unit of time by plasma (in mL/minute) flowing through the glomeruli of the kidneys.

Half-life ($t_{1/2}$)
The time it takes for one half of the original amount of a drug to be removed from the body; helps to identify the relationship between plasma drug concentration, steady state, and clearance from the body;

half-life is an important variable in determining proper dosing and frequency of administration.

Health care provider-nurse communication
The accuracy and extent to which health care providers and nurses communicate between and among themselves about patient care; the strongest predictor of patient outcomes.

Hepatic blood flow
The blood flow through the liver; drug metabolism in the liver depends on adequate hepatic blood flow.

Intrinsic activity
The ability of a drug to activate a specific receptor.

Learning deficit
The void between a patient's knowledge level and what information is needed for adherence.

Lipid-soluble drug
A drug that readily passes through cell membranes; cell membranes are composed of lipids. Small, lipid-soluble, nonionized drugs readily diffuse across cell membranes, whereas larger, water-soluble, ionized drugs do not.

Magnitude of effect
The effectiveness of a drug; relates to the concentration of the drug at the receptor site.

Medication error
"Any preventable event that may cause or lead to inappropriate medication use or patient harm while the medication is in the control of the health care professional, patient, or consumer" (CDER, 2001).

Metabolism
The body's way of changing lipid-soluble drugs by transforming them into more water-soluble compounds so they can be eliminated through the kidneys in urine.

Molecular size
The size of a molecule plays a part in drug absorption; for example, urea molecules are small and pass easily across cell membranes. In contrast, glucose molecules are rather large and do not pass easily.

Onset of action
The time it takes for a drug to begin eliciting response.

Medication orders
A directive from the health care provider on behalf of the patient for a specific drug or drugs; should include the drug name, dosage, frequency, route of administration, and administration time. Half of all preventable medication errors begin with the health care provider's orders.

Passive diffusion
Movement of drugs from higher to lower concentrations across a semipermeable membrane.

Passive reabsorption
Takes place when a drug is nonionized and still has sufficient lipid solubility to diffuse back across cell membranes from the urine into the circulation.

Peak effect
The time it takes for a drug to reach its highest effective concentration in the bloodstream.

pH
The acidity or alkalinity of a solution; both the dissolution and ionization of drugs are affected by the pH values of body solutions.

Pharmaceutical phase
The stage during which the drug enters the body in one form and changes to another form to be used.

Pharmacodynamic phase
The stage during which a drug reaches its site of action and produces an effect.

Pharmacodynamics
The study of what biologically active compounds do in the body; "what the drug does to the body."

Pharmacokinetics
The study of how the body reacts to biologically active compounds; "what the body does to the drug."

Pharmacology
The study of the mechanism of action, uses, side effects, and fate of drugs in the body.

Pharmacotherapeutics
The use of drugs to alleviate the signs and symptoms of disease, delay disease progression, cure a disease, or facilitate nondrug interventions.

Pinocytosis
The process whereby a drug is engulfed and moved across cell membranes; during pinocytosis the cell wall invaginates, forms a vacuole for drug transport, breaks off, and moves into the cell.

Plasma protein
A protein (e.g., albumin) that occupies about 6% to 7% of the blood plasma in the body; reduced plasma protein levels result in higher concentrations of unbound drug.

Polarity
The electrical charge of a cell membrane; positive, negative, or neutral.

Polypharmacy
The use of many different drugs as the result of multiple disease processes, the prescribing behaviors of health care providers, and poorly coordinated patient management.

Potency
The dosage of a drug needed to produce a specific response; potency is influenced by the drug's affin-

ity for receptors and by the body's absorptive, distributive, biotransformational, and elimination capabilities.

Prodrug
A drug that is not active until it is metabolized in the liver or other tissues.

Progesterone
A natural hormone; drug metabolism during pregnancy is heightened by the effects of progesterone.

Quality of care
The best nursing and medical care provided for a patient or a population of patients by a health care provider; collaboration between health care providers and patients improves patient outcomes.

Side effects
Any undesirable effect of a medication that is expected or anticipated to occur in a predictable percentage of patients who receive a given medication; side effects range from mild to severe.

Site of drug action
The place in the body where the drug receptor is located.

Sound-alike or look-alike names
Drugs that serve different purposes but have names that sound or look similar; the most hazardous situation occurs when medications from two different classes have sound-alike or look-alike names.

Specificity
The property of receptors that allows them to differentiate among similar drugs and bind only to those with the critical features.

Steady state
The physiologic plateau in which the amount of drug eliminated from the body is equal to the amount of drug absorbed with each dose.

Tablet-splitting
The practice of cutting tablets in half to extend a prescription longer than it was originally intended or to obtain a smaller dosage of medication.

Teratogen
Any drug or compound interfering with embryonic and/or fetal development.

Timing of drug exposure
The stage of pregnancy during which the fetus is exposed to a drug taken by the mother; the fetus is most vulnerable to harm from drug exposure during the first trimester.

Total body water
All water found within the body.

Urinary pH
Describes the acidity or alkalinity of the urine; drug elimination is affected by urinary pH, because some

drugs are more readily eliminated in acid urine, but others require more basic urine.

Uterine-placental blood flow
Circulation of blood through the uterus to the placenta; optimal uterine-placental blood flow is obtained with the patient in a right or left lateral recumbent or sitting position. Any maternal position that does not optimize uterine blood flow decreases the potential for fetal drug exposure.

Verbal orders
Orders spoken aloud in person or by telephone; these orders provide more room for error than written orders or orders sent electronically.

Index

A

Abbreviations used in drug orders, 38
Absorption, drug
  in children, 43-44
  fetal-placental, 60
  food and, 68
  in older adults, 52
  during pregnancy, 59-60
  principles, 15-16
Acetaminophen (Tylenol), 1
Acetylsalicylic acid, 1
Active ingredients, 15
Active metabolites, 17
Active transport, 16, 17
Adenosine triphosphate (ATP), 16
Administration, drug, 7-13
  parenteral versus enteral, 15
Advil, 2
African Americans, 68-69
Albumin, 44, 60, 61
American Academy of Pediatrics (AAP), 62
Amulets, 70
Antacids, 29
Antagonists, 30, 32
Asian Americans, 69-70
Aspirin (Bufferin), 1

B

Bioavailability, 29
Body surface area (BSA), 43
Brand name drugs, 2
Breast milk, 62
Brown bag sessions, 51, 55
Bufferin, 1

C

Cardiac output in older adults, 52
Chemical names, 1
Cherokee Indians, 70
Children and medications
  absorption, 43-44
  body surface area (BSA) of, 43
  breast milk and, 62
  distribution, 44
  elimination, 45
  metabolism, 44-45
Christian Scientists, 70
Collaboration among health care providers, 67, 75
Costs, drug therapy, 71, 77
Coumadin, 68
Creatinine, 23

Creatinine clearance (CL), 23
Cultural beliefs
  African Americans, 68-69
  Asian Americans, 69-70
  dietary practices and, 68
  drug use and misuse and, 70
  ethnopharmacology and, 67-72
  family support networks and, 71
  Hispanic Americans, 69, 75
  language differences and, 70-71
  Native Americans, 70
  nonadherence and, 74, 77-78
  religion and, 70
  white Americans, 68
Curandero, 69
Cytochrome P 450 enzyme system activity, 44, 53

D

Decongestants, 29
Deficits, learning, 71
Deltasone, 1
Demerol, 1
Diazepam (Valium), 1
Dietary practices and cultural beliefs, 68
Dilantin, 55, 56
Diphenhydramine, 30
Distribution, drug
  in children, 44
  fetal-placental, 60-61
  in older adults, 52
  during pregnancy, 60
Documentation, drug administration, 8
Dosing
  accuracy, 7
  curve, 24, 28
  medication errors and, 38-39
Drugs
  absorption, 15-16
  active ingredients, 15
  administration route, 8
  brand or trade names, 2
  cost of, 71, 77
  distribution, 16
  documentation, 8
  elimination, 17
  enteral, 15
  exposure timing, 62
  formulations, 15
  generic, 1, 71
  half-lives, 23, 60
  interactions with food, 68

Neurotransmitters, 29
Nonadherence by patients, 74, 77-78
Norepinephrine, 30
Nuprin, 2
Nutrient absorption, 68

O

Older adults and medications
    absorption, 52
    distribution, 52
    elimination, 53
    metabolism, 52-53
    polypharmacy and, 51, 55, 56
Ondansteron (Zofran), 37
Onset of action, 23
Oral medications
    children and, 43-44
    dosing errors and, 38-39
Orders, medication, 37-38
Outcomes, patient, 37, 72
Over the counter drugs (OTC), 51, 68

P

Parenteral drugs, 15
    children and, 44
Passive diffusion, 16
Passive reabsorption, 17
Patients
    cultural beliefs of, 67-72
    education, 71-72, 77-78
    identification, 7-8
    literacy, 71
    nonadherence, 74, 77-78
    outcomes, 37
    right to refuse drugs, 8
Peak effect, 23
Pharmaceutic phase of drug activity, 15
Pharmacodynamics
    in children, 45
    during pregnancy, 61-62
    principles, 29-30
Pharmacokinetic phase of drug activity, 15-17
    pregnancy and, 59-60
Phenytoin (Dilantin), 55, 56
Ph of body solutions, 16, 59
Pinocytosis, 16
Plasma proteins, 44, 52, 61
Polarity of drug molecules, 16
Polypharmacy, 51, 55, 56
Potency, 30, 32
Prednisone (Deltasone), 1
Pregnancy, medication use in
    absorption and, 59-60
    distribution and, 60
    elimination and, 60
    fetal-placental considerations of, 60-61, 63-64
    metabolism and, 60
    pharmacodynamic considerations of, 61-62
    pharmacokinetic considerations of, 59-60

Prodrugs, 17
Progesterone, 60
Propranolol, 30

Q

Q-Profen, 2

R

Receptors, 29-30
Refuse, right to, 8
Religious beliefs, 70
Route, drug administration, 8
    children and, 43-44

S

Schedules, drug administration, 8
Self-treatment, 68-70
Side effects, drug, 51
Steady state, 23
Support networks, family, 71
Sweat lodges, 70

T

Tablet splitting, 39
Teratogens, 61-62
Thousand-year eggs, 70
Tiger balm, 70
Timing of drug exposure, 62
Topical medications, 44
Toxic metabolites, 17
Trade name drugs, 2
Tylenol, 1

U

Umbilical cord blood flow, 61
United States Adopted Name (USAN) Council, 1
United States Pharmacopeia/National Formulary (USP-NF), 2
Uterine-placental blood flow, 60-61

V

Valium, 1
Verbal orders, 38
Vitamin supplements, 68
Voodoo practitioners, 69

W

Warfarin (Coumadin), 68
Water, body
    in children, 43
    in older adults, 52, 54
    during pregnancy, 59
White Americans, 68
White flower, 70

Y

Yin and yang, 69

Z

Zofran, 37

English/Spanish Common Medical Terms

Introductory		Does it hurt when I press here?	¿Le duele cuando aprieto aquí?
My name is _____.	Me llamo _____.	Here, There.	Aquí, Ahi.
What is your name?	¿Cómo se llama usted?	**The Body**	
Do you speak English?	¿Habla ingles?	Abdomen	El abdomen
Yes, No.	Sí, No.	Ankle	El tobillo
I would like to examine you now.	Quisiera examinarlo(a) ahora.	Arm	El brazo
General		Back	La espalda
How do you feel?	¿Cómo se siente?	Bones	Los huesos
Good (fine)	Bien	Chest	El pecho
Bad	Mal	Ears	Los oídos
Better	Mejor	Elbow	El codo
Worse	Peor	Eye	El ojo
Are you allergic to anything?	¿Tiene usted algerias?	Face	La cara
Medications, foods, insect bites?	¿Medicinas, alimentos, picaduras de insectos?	Finger	El dedo
Do you take any medications?	¿Toma usted algunas medicinas?	Foot	El pie
Do you have a history of	¿Padece usted enfermedad	Hand	La mano
Heart disease?	del corazón?	Head	La cabeza
Diabetes?	del diabetes?	Hip	La cadera
Epilepsy?	de la epilepsia?	Knee	La rodilla
Bronchitis?	de bronquitis?	Leg	La pierna
Emphysema?	de enfesema?	Lip	El labio
Asthma?	de asma?	Mouth	La boca
Pain		Muscles	Los músculos
Have you any pain?	¿Tiene dolor?	Neck	El cuello
Where is the pain?	¿Dónde está el dolor?	Nose	La naríz
Do you have any pain here?	¿Tiene usted dolor aquí?	Penis	El pene, el miembro
How severe is the pain?	¿Qué tan fuerte es el dolor?	Shoulder	El hombro
Mild, moderate, sharp, or severe?	¿Ligero, moderado, agudo, severo?	Stomach	El estómago, la panza, la barriga
What were you doing when the pain started?	¿Qué hacía usted cuando le comenzó el dolor?	Tongue	La lengua
Have you ever had this pain before?	¿Ha tenido este dolor antes? (¿Ha sido siempre así?)	Thigh	El muslo
Do you have a pain in your side?	¿Tiene usted dolor en el costado?	Vagina	La vagina
Is it worse now?	¿Está peor ahora?	**Organs**	
Does it still pain you?	¿Le duele todavía?	Brain	El cerebro
Did you feel much pain at the time?	¿Sintió mucho dolor entonces?	Heart	El corazón
Show me where.	Muéstreme dónde.	Intestines/bowels	Los intestinos/las entrañas
		Kidney	El riñón
		Liver	El hígado
		Lungs	Los pulmones

Modified from Ignatavicius DD, Workman ML: *Medical-surgical nursing: critical thinking for collaborative care*, ed 5, St. Louis, 2006, Saunders; and Lewis SL, et al: *Clinical companion to medical-surgical nursing*, ed 7, St. Louis, 2007, Mosby.